Propose 2 Days/week   2, 8, 9, 19, 20   Evaluations
300 days x 2/week 600   111 - 113 -
48 weeks

Look up The Jane's Mission, Vision and Values

P 41 becoming Part of the care team

Address Care givers, Families   (step 6)

5/29 emailed Robin
Re: Other Programs

Call Jenifer or DANA
or Email

48   30
6   15
48   440
28,200   28,640
9440
10/week supplies

Enclose Evaluations

Artists-In-Residence

The Creative Center's Approach to Arts in Healthcare

Geraldine Herbert
Jane Waggoner Deschner
Robin Glazer

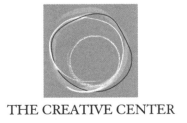

THE CREATIVE CENTER

Funding to develop this book, generously given by

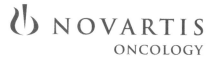 NOVARTIS
ONCOLOGY

ISBN 0-9778862-0-4

Distributed by The Creative Center
147 West 26th Street, 6th Floor
New York, NY 10001
646-336-7612
info@thecreativecenter.org
www.thecreativecenter.org

Cover artwork by Suzanne Thacher

Graphic design by Jane Waggoner Deschner, MFA

Printed by Artcraft Printers, Billings, Montana

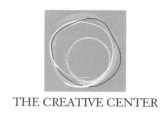

THE CREATIVE CENTER

*Dedicated to the creative spirit
found in all of us.*

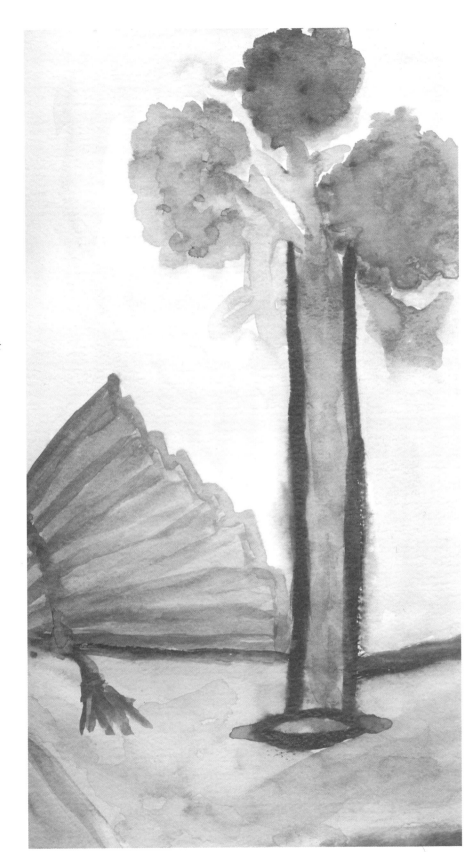

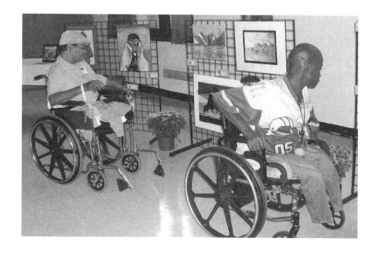

Table of Contents

Caring for Caregivers: What Can an AIR Do?
How AIRs Care for Themselves
Caregiving Takes the Efforts of Many

Appendices

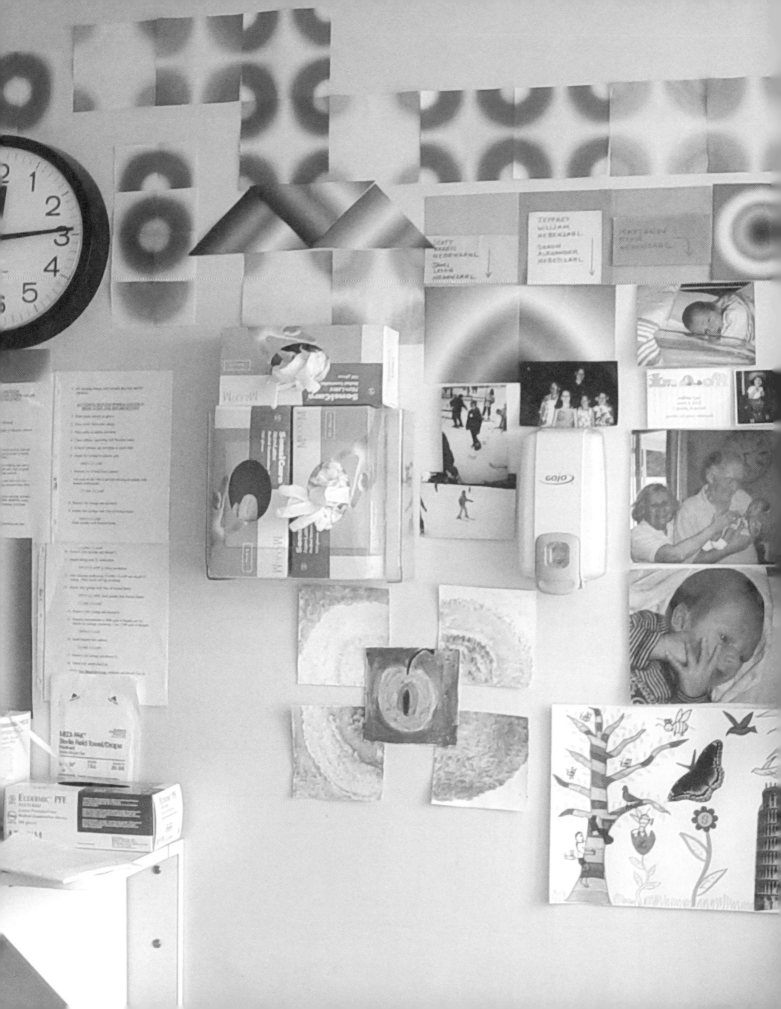

Introduction

If you believe that art is good, then it is good everywhere, and especially good in places where the human spirit is in need. We have written this book with the hope that it will enable *more artists* to make *more art* with *more people* in *more hospitals*.

Art — In a Healthcare Setting?

Who wants to make art when they are sick? It turns out a large majority of people do. Isn't artmaking intrusive and out-of-place in a hospital; and don't the doctors and nurses find that the artist gets in the way? Artists that are respectful, kind and creative are always welcomed; and the overwhelmed doctors and nurses are often overjoyed that patients are engaged in something that takes their minds off their pain and anxiety.

What we really want to know is why do patients and their families respond so fully to the opportunity to make art when they are hospitalized? Certainly part of the answer lies in the culture of most healthcare institutions. In order to "treat" a person, medical personnel often need to divest patients of their autonomy. The abilities to choose, to maintain privacy, to retain the day-to-day individuality that describes each one of us is often lost when we put on a hospital gown. Many patients are hospitalized for long periods of time, enveloped by boredom which breeds anxiety and filled with a fear which can become pervasive. Patients who are in pain need medication — they also need people and companionship and creativity.

The Creative Center learned a lot about the value of art and artmaking when we did a study of patient and staff response to The Center's Artist-In-Residence Program in five New York City hospitals. We learned that in working with our artists, many people were making art for the first time and they took enormous pride in what they had made — families treasured the patients' work and often returned to the hospital to claim it. We learned that doctors and nurses thought that patients were better able to discuss and to make treatment choices after they had made art. And, we learned that our belief that *medicine may cure the body, but art heals the spirit* was indeed true.

How Our Program Works

Artists-In-Residence (AIRs) give people the opportunity, the freedom, to make art that is truthful to the spirit of the maker — supporting, encouraging and enabling people with life-threatening illnesses to discover and explore their own voice, their own brush stroke, dance step or poetic line. Because making art has something to do with overcoming things, the obstacles, idiosyncracies and challenges that must be faced in doing one's own artwork become a source of strength and self-discovery.

What The Creative Center artists frequently hear is that the diagnosis of cancer or another life-threatening illness diminishes and often entirely depletes people of who they used to know themselves to be. Their individuality is often no longer visible; it may not be commented upon, encouraged or valued by others who now see them only as patients, unwell spouses or parents — or heart-breakingly sick children.

When a young woman tapes a watercolor to the wall of her hospital room, or a child hands his doctor a lumpy clay elephant, or an elderly man recites a line of poetry, they reveal their individuality to the hospital staff. They are not the bone cancer patient in Bed 309, they are creative children and adults whose spirits are thriving in the face of tremendous physical challenges. Their art tells us so.

What Kind of a Book Is This?

Artists-In-Residence: The Creative Center's Approach to Arts in Healthcare describes, explains, examines, persuades and proselytizes about our time-tested, continually honed approach to artists working with patients and caregivers in healthcare settings. Artist-In-Residence programs exist in other places and are done in many ways. This book is all about what we have found works for us and how; it is not meant to be a definitive study or overview of the field.

Using This Book

Within these pages you will read two different kinds of texts, each type-set in its own way. The first, printed in an italic, non-serif font, is comprised of excerpts from our Creative Center AIRs' logs. After each day spent working at the hospital, artists are required to journal about their experiences — how the day went; whom they worked with; the art that was made and/or conversations that transpired; interactions they had with staff and families — and how they felt about it. Each month, artists turn their log entries into The Center; in return, they receive a paycheck. The logs, an important part of the AIR experience, are archived and were excerpted throughout this book to illustrate, in the words of only those who have truly done the work can, what amazing experiences can transpire. All names, places and any detail that might be used to identify the patient, family or healthcare institution have been changed.

The second kind of text you will encounter is serifed and not italic. Here we articulate, more didactically, the concepts the adjacent logs are illustrating. Reading the two kinds of texts together presents the intellectual and the emotional approaches, both the thinking-about-the-process and the doing-with-the-patient. The photographs were taken by our Artists-In-Residence during the course of their daily work. Please read the section about our AIRs — they are exceptional individuals.

We suggest that first you read the book from front to back; the chapters build upon one another. Chapters 2–4 give the reader a very basic introduction to the partners — what it is to be an artist, a healthcare institution and a patient in the context of our artmaking in healthcare work. Chapters 5–7 discuss the ways these partners work with one another — how The Creative Center trains our artists; ways of understanding and working within

that unique culture of a healthcare institution; and the experience of making art with patients. Chapter 8 explains the portable studio — how the artist creates an art studio at a patient's bedside, as well as suggested media, materials, methods and ideas for projects. Chapters 9–10 discuss additional aspects that are important for an AIR to understand — caregivers and caregiving, and working with the dying. Chapters 11–13 return to the nuts and bolts of beginning, establishing, marketing and maintaining a program — why The Creative Center came to be who we are and how we do the things we do today.

The Appendices complement and add to the book. You will find further information about the field and The Creative Center's work; a sample release form; more ways to use other art media in the hospital; a brief explanation of the systems of the human body and some life-threatening illnesses; our favorite resources; and a glossary. The glossary gives definitions of terms and explanations of concepts that may not be familiar to the reader, as well as how these are used particularly in the Arts in Healthcare field. This book may not answer all your questions, but after reading these pages, you will now know what and whom to ask.

If You Are...

If you are an artist, you know how making art can capture your attention, your imagination — your very being; that it can transport you to another time and place, and leave you with the desire to have that experience all over again. *If you are a patient,* you know how valuable those times are when you forget to think about your illness, and how you wish that you could create tangible things that reflect the spirit and the hope within you. *If you are a healthcare administrator, a physician, a nurse or social worker,* you may have witnessed the small miracles that occur when artist and patient make art together. It is our hope that this book will enable artists, patients and healthcare staff to discover the many ways that art can transform our medical environments and the people who rely on these places to make them well.

Use this book, and all you find within, as an inspiration and resource to pursue your creative vision. The Creative Center is here to assist you in all the ways that we can.

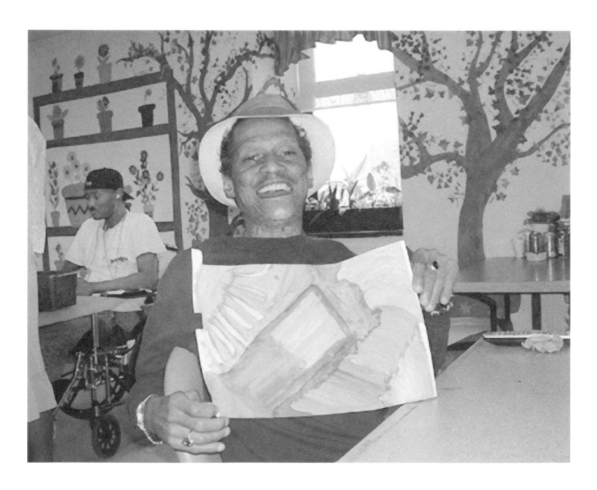

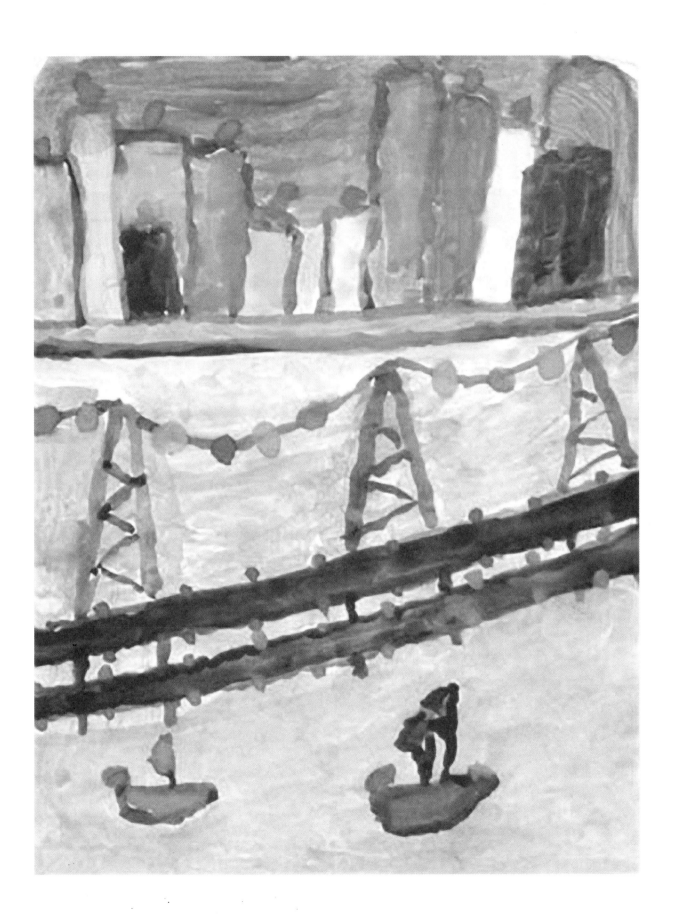

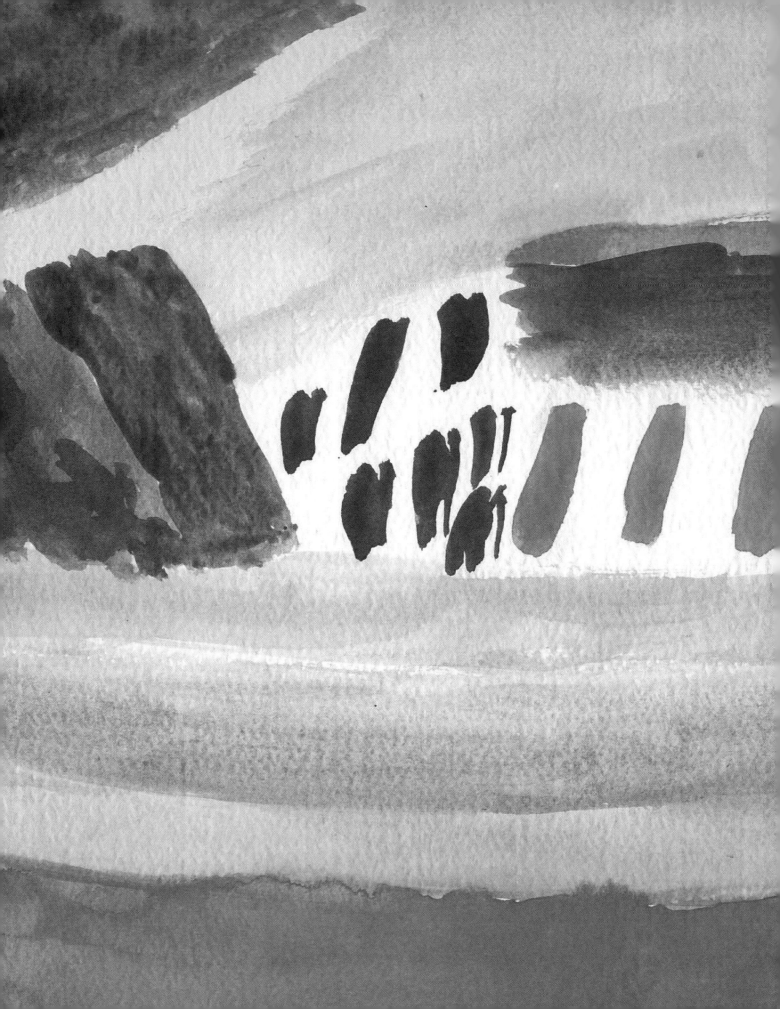

Being an Artist

I realized today how dramatically different the time I spend at the hospital is from the time I spend in my studio. When I'm sitting with a patient, my time is theirs completely: they determine, in large part, the pace at which we work, the subject matter of our conversation, the mood, the duration. I am there for them and so I dismiss my typical drives to work fast, to be focused on the outcome of my labor, to strive toward some finished product.

In an almost Zen-like fashion, when in the hospital, I give myself over to whatever scenario presents itself; I remain extremely alert to the needs of the patient, do my best to react in whatever way will yield for them the most comfort, and allow myself to be guided by them and the situation. It is, I guess, a more reactive state as opposed to the mode in which I normally work, for myself, satisfying my own needs as an artmaker.

Artists are often described as unconventional and individualistic, curious and questioning, driven to create, highly sensitive. Artists take familiar words, materials or ideas and combine them in new ways, creating something unique — a painting, song or story that has never existed quite in this way before. They are comfortable with risk; they think "outside the box." For many it is a difficult life, one they wouldn't have chosen, but can't abandon as it is an integral part of who they are.

Many artists consider the work they do in the community around them as a significant part of their artistic practice. Some teach children; some donate original artworks to worthy causes; some use their art to advocate politically; others work with patients and caregivers in hospitals.

Qualities of an Effective AIR

What qualities, when transferred from artist's studio to hospital bedside, facilitate an artist working successfully as an Artist-In-Residence?

- Flexibility
- Openness
- Ability to improvise and take risks
- Resourcefulness
- Playfulness
- Capacity to stay in the process
- Empathy and compassion

- Passion for art and creativity
- Altruistic attitude
- Knowledge of art history, materials and methods
- Well-developed sense of humor!

In a healthcare setting, an artist creates both art and relationships. What other qualities are important for an artist to possess?
- Desire to connect with people and give back to the community
- Passion for sharing and teaching art and artmaking
- Sensitivity to and respect for diverse cultures, biologies, physicalities and ethnicities

- Capacity to listen and be sincerely supportive
- Well-defined personal and professional boundaries
- Ability to collaborate
- Good health (no physical or mental condition that would endanger self or others in a a hospital)

Artists model creative, adapting behaviors to anxious patients and stress-filled caregivers. *Successful AIRs help people play, experiment and stay in the process.* When a patient says, "I can't; I'm not artistic!" one AIR replies, "Make something awful!" And away they go!

Rocio loves landscapes and so we begin together by drawing the view from her window in colored pencil. When we're done, we look at each other's work. Rocia taps at her heart and says, "They say you can tell a lot about a person's insides when you look at their artwork and I think it's true." I'm a little blown away by how simply she's said something I've thought for a long time, but not in nearly as clear a way. I ask her what she sees in her drawing, a delicate and well-composed picture of mostly greens and grays of the bridge, a long strip of the East River and the edge of Manhattan. "I see someone who is sad and tired," she says. I ask, "What about this part?" pointing to the bright pink and yellow and green polka dots of cars lining the FDR drive. She laughs and says she put them in because she was thinking how sad the painting looked and she wanted it to be happier. "What do you see in mine?" I ask and hear one of the nicest compliments I have ever received. "I see someone who is open," she replies.

Louis was red faced, bloated and looked uncomfortable when I saw him. He told me how his symptoms were progressing and then said, "What else do you have on that cart?" I told him about the varied materials — drawing, collage, paints, pencils, watercolor crayons, paper clay, air drying clay, origami, etc. and he asked me if I would sit so that he could draw my picture. So for two hours that afternoon I sat (and gained a greater appreciation for all the models who have sat for my artwork) and Louis drew. Unlike our other visits he spoke very little but said to me "...you are so calm. I don't know how you manage that but I thank you for bringing a bit of it here each week. You leave a piece of it with me." When he finished, he was satisfied with his work but gave it to me saying, "I don't have a use for these kinds of things anymore."

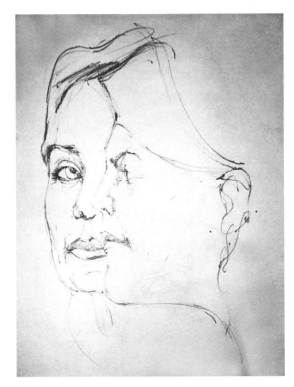

Methods and Materials

Artists who work in any medium — visual, literary or performing — can be AIRs; many choose media other than their primary ones when working with patients. One AIR says watching patients create gives her great ideas and new ways to use materials. Whatever methods and materials an artist is comfortable sharing, the people the artist is working with will be comfortable using. The artist's enthusiasm, knowledge and creative ideas will "rub off." In a hospital, art making is primarily about establishing a supportive interaction between artist and participant in order to experience the creative process.

Becoming an AIR

Not every artist is suited to working with the sick or dying. At The Creative Center, becoming employed as an AIR is a process of evaluation for both the artist and The Center.

Typically the artist first fills out an application. Promising candidates are then invited for an interview during which their personality and artistic expertise are evaluated in the context of this kind of work. This is also the artist's opportunity to ask any and all questions about rewards and difficulties. If the artist and The Center feel they are a good fit, the process of contacting references, checking background and scheduling a health screening begins. The next step is the artist's training!

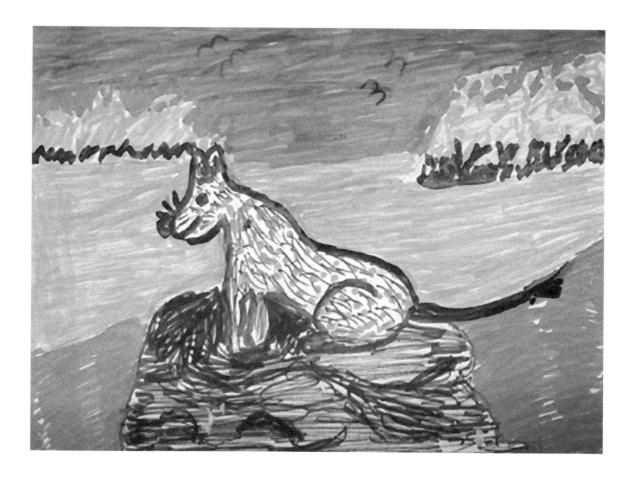

About The Creative Center's Artists-In-Residence (AIRs)

Throughout this book are excerpts from AIRs' logs and pictures they have taken in hospitals and hospices. To preserve patient and caregiver confidentiality, we are unable to credit the writers and photographers of each selection. The following exceptional AIRs have graciously allowed us to use their thoughts and images to illuminate the practices, theories and concepts in this book.

Virginia Arnold studied fine art at Colorado College and the Denver Art Academy, and painting and textile design at the New School in New York City. Her work has been exhibited in galleries in the New York area, including The Creative Center. After working for three years as an AIR at Columbia-Presbyterian, Virginia was diagnosed with cancer herself. "Art is what makes us human," says Virginia, "Sharing this process with patients gives us the strength to survive beyond illness."

Catharine Balco is an artist, teacher and Artist-In-Residence in the bone marrow transplant unit at New York Hospital. She is currently pursuing her Master of Fine Arts at the Yale School of Art. Catharine has exhibited her cityscape paintings in solo and group shows in New England and New York including recent two-person shows at the Carol Craven Gallery in Massachusetts, The Atlantic Gallery in New York City and The Brooklyn Public Library. Her awards include a Weir Farm Trust Residency Fellowship, a Yale School of Art at Norfolk Fellowship and a Vermont Community Foundation Grant. "Drawing enables us to express our shared humanity in very simple terms. I feel very grateful to have participated in drawing sessions with patients who have inspired me with their courage, humor and willingness to express themselves."

Patricia Begley was born in Ireland, where she has returned to live and write poetry. While earning her degree in literature and writing at Hunter College in New York City, she was editor of the literary magazine, *Returning Women*. She attended the Vermont Studio Center on a Writer's

Grant, won the Bernard Cohen Short Story Prize and was a Thomas W. Smith Academic Fellow.

Julia Chiang studied art history and studio art at New York University. She has been a resident at Hap Clay Studios (China), Vermont Studio Center and Henry Street Settlement. "Working at Mount Sinai has allowed me to combine my interest in making art with that of being involved with the community. People's extreme strength and willingness to try something new in such a difficult time is always amazing to me."

Ramona Candy is a dancer, teacher, designer and performer. She earned a Bachelor of Arts in Art from City College while she pursued a dance career. She danced for twenty years with the Charles Moore Dance Theater and then returned to painting and collage. Her artwork combines her Haitian heritage, her Brooklyn upbringing and elements of dance. "Creating art with patients at North General Hospital has sometimes been challenging, but it is the gentle shift in a reluctant patient, the smile of loved ones or a nod from staff that quickly snuffs my frustration."

Melissa Chapin is a mixed media artist who studied at the Art Students League of New York with Bruce

Dorfman, Knox Martin and William Scharf. She exhibits her ardor for color and the natural world in her assemblage paintings, alternative photography and collaborative artist books. She is known for leading fun, imaginative, sometimes irreverent art workshops. Since 2003, she's been an AIR at Calvary Hospital. "The exploration, expression and creative solace of even the simplest encounter continually reminds me of the grace and grit of the human spirit and the gifts of the Artist-In-Residence program. I couldn't ask for a more fulfilling experience and I'm deeply grateful to be part of The Creative Center community."

Aisha Cousins is an AIR at Brooklyn Hospital. A mixed media artist, she lives in Brooklyn, New York. A graduate of Oberlin College, Aisha studied studio art, sociology and Black history. Her mixed media series, that connect aspects of Black history to current trends in Black American culture, have been shown at Skylight Gallery, Savacou Gallery and the Museum of Contemporary Diasporian Arts. She states, "I have this theory that everyone has a certain level of artistic genius. My job is to help each patient find it. I encourage kids to trust their creative instincts, to make something new and be free. That's important for everyone, but especially for kids in the hospital. Everyone is telling them what to do. Constantly. They need freedom — it's essential."

New York University Hospital's AIR **Mare Dianora** has a Master of Fine Arts in Interdisciplinary Arts from Goddard College in Plainfield, Vermont (August 2005). Her media include correspondence art, book arts, ceramics and photography. "My work at the hospital is about creating a connection between the patient and myself. Through the process of making art, we find common ground and begin a relationship that can happen in only one session — or one that will be nurtured over many, many weeks."

Mary Didoardo is a graduate of Pratt Institute and has been a practicing painter and sculptor for over thirty-five years. She teaches in New York City Public Schools through Studio in a School and Young Audiences NY; she is an AIR at Long Island College Hospital. "In my studio, art making is an alternate process of exploration and critique. In the hospital, I meet many people as they come and go and that is one the pleasures of being an Artist-In-Residence for The Creative Center. My typical residency day involves moving around the hospital, inviting patients to choose from an assortment of materials and projects. The most common response I hear is, 'I've

never painted before.' or 'I haven't done this since I was a little girl/boy.' — often said with the intention to dismiss any idea of attempting it now. But people are full of surprises and they often say 'yes.' Sometimes their resulting drawings and paintings are a revelation to themselves!"

Karen Furth is a photographer and artist whose work has been exhibited at many galleries in New York City including A.I.R., Pulse Art and 494 Gallery. She has been involved with community programs for many years and has taught at The Times Square, a supportive program for low-income residents. "Working with patients at Lenox Hill Hospital has made me reconsider how people approach art as individuals — what they are looking for or need to find in the process of making it. As an artist, it has given me the freedom to try new materials and reminds me of why I became an artist in the first place."

Colleen Kerns earned her Bachelor of Fine Arts in Communication Design from Kutztown University, Pennsylvania. She has pursued various paths in art, illustration and design. Exhibiting in New York, Pennsylvania, Connecticut and Maryland, her most recent show, "Uptown Art Stroll" was seen in June 2005. Her preferred media include acrylic and collage. She states, "It has been very rewarding both artistically and personally to engage and challenge my patients at Zicklin Jewish Hospital Residence in the process of making art…to encourage the uniqueness of self-expression and validate their presence in the here and now."

Barbara Lewis Marco has been an AIR in hospice and palliative care since 2000. She is the author of *The Little Book of Courage, An Illustrated Guide to Challenging Our Fears.* She leads expressive arts workshops; is an arts instructor in the Narrative Medicine Program at Columbia University Medical School; and runs an art program at Columbia Presbyterian's Pediatric Neurology Clinic. "Being an AIR at Beth Israel Hospice is the most unique, creative, challenging, inspiring and rewarding experience imaginable. It may sound corny, but I don't care; I feel truly privileged to be doing it. The ideals of The Creative Center for this work are very special. Here is the clearest, most fearless intention for simple, deeply creative human interaction at times of great suffering and that is something truly rare in these times."

Joan Mellon is a painter who has a Bachelor of Fine Arts from the School of Visual Arts and a Master of Arts

from SUNY Empire State College. The materials she has used to explore her interest in color and create single and multi-panel color abstractions and works on paper are oil paint and pastels often underpainted with acrylic and watercolors. Her work is represented in the collection of the Museum of Modern Art/Franklin Furnace Archives, Johnson & Johnson, the School of Visual Arts and private collections. As an Artist-In-Residence since 2002, Joan is grateful to have had the opportunity to work with people of diverse ages and cultures at Calvary Hospital, an end-of-life care facility, and at the bedside and in the infusion suites at Roosevelt Hospital and St. Vincent Comprehensive Cancer Center.

Daniela Mizrahi is a figurative painter and native of Argentina. Her main mediums are oil painting, drawing and printmaking (woodcuts). After completing her studies in Latin American literature at the University of Buenos Aires, she came to New York to study painting. For four years she attended The Art Students League and The New York Academy of Art where she earned a Master of Fine Arts. In 1998 she began working for The Creative Center as an Artist-In-Residence, and as a drawing and painting instructor. After ten years, in 2005, she returned to her native country, where she teaches art classes at her own studio. Working with children and adults as an AIR became an intense and creative experience for her. A huge variety of art projects and ideas of how to approach the artistic process were always the main motivation (as well as a challenge) for both herself and the patients. She feels that the idea of bringing art into a hospital context is always based in trying to experience a real connection, in that specific moment, between herself and the other person. "Art is a path to reach our own identities."

Antonia Perez is a painter who combines needlework and household goods in her projects to create invented worlds. She received her training in art schools in Mexico City, Vancouver and New York and exhibits locally and nationally. "I value making art with people at Bellevue Medical Center as it offers them a means to relax while stimulating powerful self-expression."

Over the last twenty years **Mimi Quillin** has combined a performing career with choreography. She is equally at home in the commercial theatre world and the non-profit sector. Her choreography work includes TV soaps, NYC Dumbo Dance Festival, Edinburgh Fringe, two film collaborations, an artist's

residency with The Creative Center and several dramatic productions at the Flea Theater in Tribeca.

Rodger Stevens was born in Brooklyn, New York, and educated at the Parsons School of Design and The School of Visual Arts, both in New York City. His sculpture and drawings have been appearing in galleries, museums and publications in the United States and elsewhere since 1993. He has done commissioned work for such clients as The Whitney Museum of American Art, The Katonah Museum, The Bristol Museum, Tiffany & Co., Jonathan Adler, Yohji Yamamoto, The New York Children's Museum of Art, The Federal Reserve Bank of New York and MTV. But probably the most rewarding

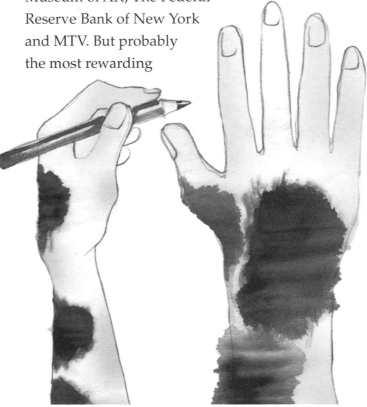

thing Rodger has done with his passion is share it with the patients he sees every week at New York Hospital and Terrence Cardinal Cooke Healthcare Center.

Ellen Wallenstein earned a Bachelor of Arts in Art History at SUNY Stony Brook (1974) and a Master of Fine Arts in Photography from Pratt Institute (1978). She has also studied at the Visual Studies Workshop and Center for Book Arts. The mediums she employs include photography, collage, stamp art and book art. Her most recent exhibition (January 2006) was part of a group show "I Bienal de Arte Contemporaneo," sponsored by Fundacion Once at the Circula de Bellas Artes in Madrid, Spain. Other exhibitions include Center for Book Arts, New York City, Ellis Island Museum, Brooklyn Museum, Visual Arts Gallery, Harpercollins Exhibition Space and Camera Club of New York. Ellen, an AIR at Englewood Hospital, says, "The best thing a patient said to me was 'You made my pain go away.'"

David Wander studied at Rhode Island School of Design and Pratt Institute in New York. He works in many mediums and is currently exhibiting large oil paintings and pastels. "My work has allowed me to bring my enthusiasm for the creative process into hospital rooms, drawing and painting with the people at Beth Israel Cardiology."

Neil Whitacre grew up in Iowa and was educated in Milwaukee, Wisconsin. His large, highly detailed pen and ink drawings are based on personal experiences. In 2005, he showed work in Miami, New York, Houston, Chicago, Portland, Toronto, Paris, Tokyo and Turin, Italy; he is represented by Richard Heller Gallery in Los Angeles. Neil writes, "My work with The Creative Center at New York Hospital is the most life affirming and inspiring thing I do."

Eileen T. Wold earned her Bachelor of Fine Arts at Loyola College and studied for one year at the Art Academy in Leuven, Belgium. Eileen has exhibited her work at New York galleries including Art Gotham, Blue Sky Gallery, Gallery 402 and Tribute Art Gallery. Her works in oil explore themes in landscape, ranging from the subtle properties of the horizon to the industrial atmosphere of the American smokestack. In 2005, she was the Artist-In-Residence at The Terrence Cardinal Cooke Healthcare Center in New York City, where she worked with over thirty residents diagnosed with AIDS and cancer or on dialysis. She organized an art exhibit that highlighted fifteen of her most accomplished artists.

Being a Healthcare Institution

Artists-In-Residence work most commonly in hospitals and hospices, places a healthy person has little reason to know much about. A rudimentary understanding of types of healthcare institutions, their employees and volunteers, and their regulatory practices will help artists adapt to this specialized environment.

The Business of Being a Hospital

Basically, a hospital is an institution whose primary function, according to the American Hospital Association, is to provide diagnostic and treatment services for patients who have a variety of medical conditions. These are categorized as surgical, non-surgical, rehabilitative or psychiatric.

The most common type of hospital, *general hospitals*, treat a wide range of diseases and injuries. Usually the major healthcare facility in an area, these institutions have an emergency department, intensive care unit and specialized facilities for surgery and childbirth. The largest general hospitals are usually called medical centers and offer treatment in virtually all areas of modern medicine. *Specialized hospitals*, as their name implies, limit themselves to specialized care — some examples are cancer, trauma, children, psychiatric, rehabilitation and geriatric.

One indicator used to measure the size of a hospital is the number of staffed patient beds. New York-Presbyterian Hospital in New York City staffs over 2,100 beds; North Logan Mercy Hospital in Paris, Arkansas, 16. Staffed beds are used for *routine care* in general medical-surgical cases or *special care* as in intensive care or coronary care units.

There are over 7,500 hospitals nationwide, treating over a half million in-patients daily. Each is a business and is set up in one of three ways — non-profit, for-profit or by some level of government. A *non-profit hospital*, organized as a non-profit corporation, is often affiliated with a religious denomination. *For-profit hospitals* are investor-owned chains whose goal is to operate at a profit. *Government-owned hospitals* include city and county hospitals, those at state universities, and federal ones such as those operated by the Department of Veterans Affairs. Fundamentally, a hospital is a business and each is run with a close eye to the bottom line. Problems with rising costs, staffing shortages and medical reimbursement policies are forcing hospitals to become increasingly competitive and bottom-line oriented.

Hospice, Specialized Healthcare

Hospices provide palliative care — care that improves quality of life and manages pain rather than tries to cure a disease. Hospice care is provided in a freestanding specialized facility, in the dying patient's home or, less commonly, within a regular hospital.

Healthcare Workers & Volunteers

In 2003, over six million people nationwide worked in hospitals providing direct patient care services: registered nurses; licensed practical and licensed vocational nurses, aides (nursing, psychiatric and home health); occupational, respiratory and physical therapists; social workers; and physicians and surgeons.

Teamwork is an important aspect of patient care in both hospital and hospice settings; each healthcare worker from physician to aide has an important role to play in caring for the patient. The Artist-In-Residence who becomes part of that team soon realizes that a hierarchy often exits.

Hospital and hospice volunteers perform many valuable ancillary services and are organized and administered through each institution's volunteer services program. Generally volunteers are senior citizens or students. AIRs often attend the volunteer orientation and training program to gain basic familiarity with the hospital in which they will be working.

Then the doctor (who Deb had been wanting to talk to) and two medical students came in so she and I said our goodbyes. Later the physician stopped me in the hall and thanked me for visiting Deb. He said that family and friends seemed to be pulling away from her as she was declining. He hadn't seen her previous artwork but said he was glad to see her talking with me when he arrived.

This morning I spent ages picking out flowers and fruit for today's still life. Eventually I decided on bright Gerbera daisies, goldenrod, lemons and limes to complement a new straw hat and gauzy, hand-dyed scarf. I spent some extra time setting up, not only adding a seashell but also organizing the storage shelf and cart since JCAHO is due tomorrow.

The Joint Commission on Accreditation of Healthcare Organizations

One cannot spend much time in a hospital before hearing the words "Joint Commission" or "Jayco." The Joint Commission on Accreditation of Healthcare Organizations (JCAHO) is a powerful entity. An independent, not-for-profit organization, established more than fifty years ago, it sets the standards by which healthcare quality is measured in America and around the world. Joint Commission accreditation means an institution has voluntarily sought evaluation and met stringent national health and safety standards. Learning that Jayco is coming causes everyone employed by a healthcare institution to scurry frantically to make certain that everything meets requirements and follows regulations. (A regulation can be as simple as requiring that no boxes be stored on the floor or under a desk or as complex as infection control protocols.)

JCAHO recognizes that the needs of patients extend beyond purely physical care, to include the mind and spirit. Recent JCAHO Environment of Care (EC) standards suggest incorporating the arts by stipulating that:

- the hospital establish an environment that meets the needs of patients, encourages a positive self-image, and respects their human dignity. (EC 3.1)
- the built environment support the development and maintenance of the patient's interests, skills, and opportunities for personal growth. (EC 3.4)

Examples cited include art exhibits, musical performances, access to nature, and opportunities for social interaction among patients through recreational interchange. The examples call for hospitals to make adequate arrangements for patients' leisure-time activities that consider and respond to their needs.

Earlier in the morning Sarah, the social worker, had mentioned a young woman who was very depressed and who she hoped would do something with me. Chelsea is 37 and has two children — 1 who's 16 and another 12 — a single mother in extreme pain and juggling too many things. When I met her she was in great pain but she wanted to hear me out and talk. She told me she likes Bob Ross paintings!

At first she said no...she was in too much pain to do anything even though she likes to paint. I told her that sometimes making something distracts people enough to concentrate on something else rather than on the pain. She asked me to come up with a project that would be very tedious and would take a lot of detail and concentration to keep her mind busy. I suggested cutting intricate shapes to form a collage.

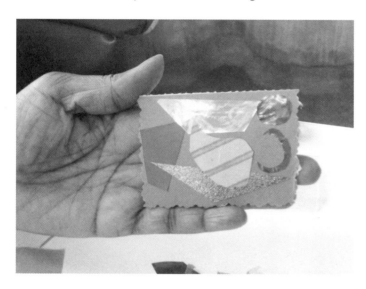

We got working and she worked very slowly and carefully, talking to me the entire time. She was very anxious and worried about her illness — still not sure what form of cancer she had and in so much pain.

A doctor came in to talk with her but she insisted I stay. She actually asked him if he could return later because she wanted to focus on her art. I think it hurt too much for her to focus on her illness.

Utilizing the Arts in the Hospital

No matter the size, type or method of organization, hospitals are businesses and must run cost-effectively to stay open. The enlightened hospital administrator knows that utilizing the arts is one way growing numbers of hospitals are not only helping their patients, but also differentiating themselves from their competitors.

A visit from an Artist-In-Residence is a sure-fire way to enhance the patient care experience. The arts in various forms (including healing gardens, artworks on walls, AIRs, musical performances) add substantially to the institution's healing environment for patients, families and staff. Providing optimal patient experiences attracts more patients; creating a healing environment improves patient care quality and helps retain staff.

Being a Patient

This is Karen's second time in two years being treated for cancer, and she is very angry. She gave up cocaine the first time around; she gave up alcohol too, and now she has to give up cigarettes. She feels victimized by cancer, and her whole life revolves around dealing with it. Her anger is like an eighteen-wheel truck — big, powerful, loud — and it is isolating her; she yells at the nurses and doctors at any given opportunity. Her family and friends, who she perceives as weak and therefore intolerable, are frightened and frozen by her outbursts.

While Karen talked, I found it tempting to jump in and deny or protest something or other that she said. But, instead, I sat and listened. I had a gut feeling that no one had done that so far and I was right; everyone was far too busy pushing her to get well.

Entering the hospital to be treated for an illness or injury begins an individual's transformation from "person" to "patient." The individual often feels isolated and frightened, having little ability to control circumstances or events. Shorter hospital stays make it difficult for patients and staff to build rapport. Patients come to welcome any opportunity that normalizes their days.

How It Feels to Be a Patient

Patients feel vulnerable; decisions involving their bodies and treatments slip from their control. A patient's sense of individuality is lost when she is identified as "the breast cancer in Room 104." A patient forfeits his privacy as healthcare staff enters the room at all hours of the day and night to prick and prod — blood is taken; medications and chemotherapy given; bodily functions are monitored; excretions are measured. The drama unfolding in the next bed is overheard; the pain and death of others are witnessed.

Patients often experience:
- Pain — its proper or improper monitoring and control.
- Discomfort — from nausea, the insertion of tubes and lines.
- Thirst or hunger — when allowed nothing by mouth (NPO).
- Fear and anxiety — about their

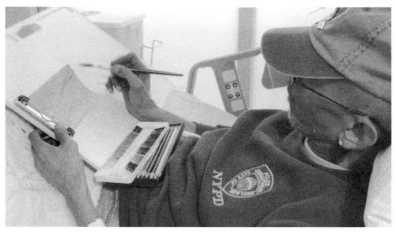

health, treatment, job, family.

- Sleep deprivation — if awakened at all times of the day and night.
- Noise — of televisions, roommates, hallways, overhead intercoms.
- Endless waiting — for nurses, doctors, tests, escorts, transfers, visits and answers.
- Nurses — who can be inattentive due to overwork and short-staffing.
- Doctors — who may also be overworked, lack empathy, give short answers to complicated questions; whose timing and delivery of "bad news" is frequently not the best.

What Kinds of Patients Will an AIR Encounter?

In healthcare settings we meet people of every age, socio-economic status, race, sexual orientation, ethnicity, educational level and religion; and people who learn and think differently than we do. We encounter patients with varying degrees of acceptance,

understanding and ability to cope with their diagnoses. We also meet people with mental, emotional and physical differences:

- Depression or anxiety.
- Drug-induced psychosis.
- Cancers — visually expressed as tumors or skin discolorations.
- Side effects from treatment — hair loss, severe weight loss, extreme swelling in different areas of the body, nausea, neutropenia, neuropathy.
- Deafness, blindness.
- Previous stroke — partial or full paralysis, aphasia.

The AIR's Focus

As AIRs, it is important to focus on what it is that those we meet have in common:

- A diagnosis.
- A form of treatment.
- A journey.
- An identity other than "patient."

Each patient is experiencing a major health crisis that is turning that person's world upside down. Many are confronting their mortality for the first time. They are searching for the cause, the cure and most importantly — for the meaning. An AIR comes to the bedside to make art — to facilitate a creative experience — not just with the patient-side of that individual, but with the person as a whole.

A Generous Spirit

Valdis Kupris lived his beliefs. While working for nearly forty years as an art professor at New York Institute of Technology, his strong and generous spirit took him many times to Latvia in Eastern Europe. When he was only six years old, he and his family fled their homeland to Germany to escape the Russians. When he was ten, they immigrated to the United States. From 1986 until his death in 2004, as soon as classes ended, he was on a plane to Latvia — returning only in time for the first day of the next semester. For the last twelve years of his life, he was intimately involved with an orphanage in Riga. He taught these children to fish and swim at summer camp; he took them to cultural events. To provide the children with histories, he took a photo of each one, every year. He said children were his angels; they were instantly comfortable in his presence.

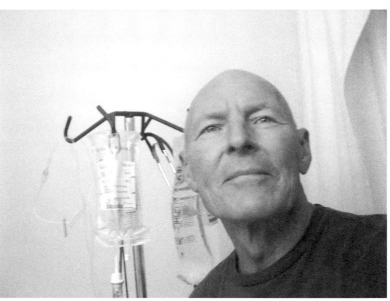

Valdis Kupris

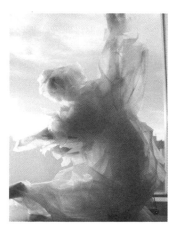

Originally a painter and sculptor, Valdis turned to working in video and photography in the early 1980s. Making a studio in his isolation room on the bone marrow transplant unit, he used his time there creatively. He photographed his hospital experience; he sculpted an angel from hospital tape; he made a lasting impression on an AIR, a group of sick children and a long-time hospital social worker. The Creative Center Artist-In-Residence (AIR) first met Valdis Kupris while he was receiving a bone marrow transplant for non-Hodgkin's lymphoma.

The following excerpts are from the log entries the AIR wrote during Valdis' first hospitalization on the bone marrow transplant unit:

September 12: *Dr. Johnson, the Director of the Bone Marrow Transplant Unit, told me to go meet Valdis Kupris, one of his patients — an artist, a painter, a photographer. There he was, surrounded by photos of the doctors, nurses, social workers, family — and his paintings, as well. He has a computer and printer in his room and he's recording his stay at the hospital. He is an amazing person. And, energy wise, he is doing great. He was sitting up and working at all times. It was amazing to meet him; we talked forever.*

September 16: *I started my day with Valdis and almost ended there as well. We worked for more than three hours. He showed me a lot of his computer work. We talked about his art. Later I showed him my paintings and we discussed them. The conversation went on and on. We talked about his illness, his strong family, his volunteer work in Latvia where he is from. About teaching and art, about mental illness and art. He was so interesting.*

September 27: *I spent more than an hour working with Valdis. We looked at more of his work. He told me interesting stories about his art career, of traveling to Africa to cast a real elephant. He was very open to the things The Creative Center does.*

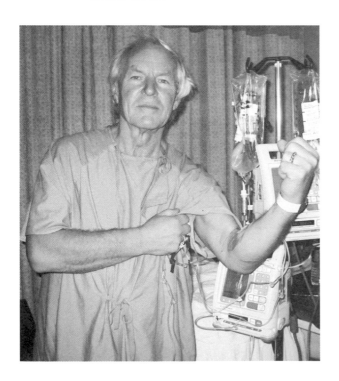

And, from his final hospitalization a few months later:

April 6: *Valdis had a lot of energy today. He has ideas and projects in mind and he was telling me all about them.*

April 16: *I had a long conversation with Valdis. He was still in the hospital and getting really tired of it.*

April 20: *I went to Valdis' room and we went for a walk. It was lovely. He told me how he taught art at New York Institute of Technology. He wanted to give me his teaching position. He was so generous with me.*

May 7: Today I arrived at the hospital and learned that Valdis was in the ICU, that he was not going to make it. I went down to the ICU. He was awake and conscious. His eyes, wide open. He was there by himself. The first thing he said to me was that the doctors told him to put his things in order, that he had days, maybe not even a week. He could not believe it. He asked them not to tell his family. His body was swollen as a balloon. But his eyes were big and shiny. He told me all the things he wanted to give me. He told me that life was unique, beautiful…I was there for an hour and a half. It was hard to be there, but it was true, very true what was happening and I saw him dying. I said I would come back later, at the end of the day. It was the end of the day for me and I went back to see Valdis. He was now with all his family. His daughters, sister and brother. He looked tired, more tired than this morning. I stayed a little while and then left.

May 14: I went directly to the ICU to see Valdis. He was not there anymore. He had passed away. I tried to find out more from the nurses. I just wanted to talk with someone and tell them I was a friend. I felt very sad, very sad and angry.

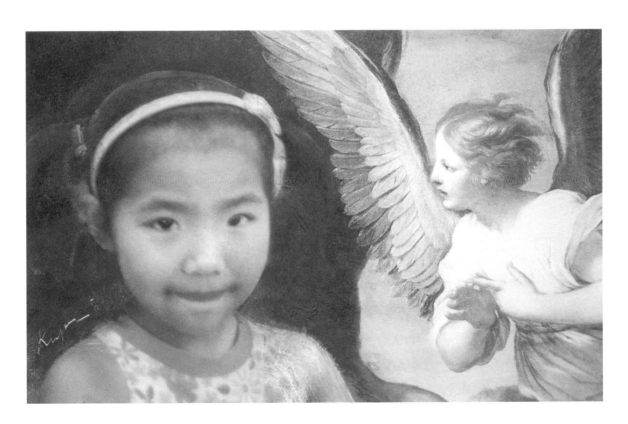

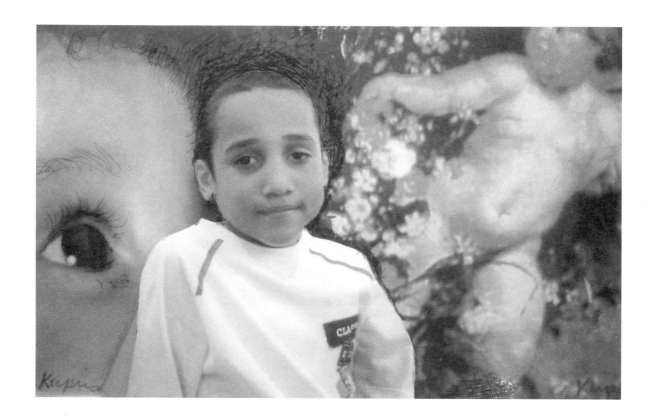

The AIR who kept these logs worked
two days a week at this hospital, on
the bone marrow transplant unit and
also downstairs with the children. On
Valdis' birthday, it had been her day
with the children. She told them about
her special artist-friend upstairs and
asked them to make birthday cards
for him — she would personally
deliver them. By now, the AIR was
well aware of Valdis' deep connection
with children. He was so touched by
their cards that he asked the AIR to go
back downstairs and take pictures of

each child with his camera. He
returned their loving gesture with
one of his own — on his computer,
he collaged a photo of each child
into images of angels, adding touches
with his own hand in ink and paint —
making every one a card which the
AIR then delivered back to the
children. The social worker in
charge of the transplant unit said it
was one of the most touching things
she had witnessed in all her years
at the hospital.

The Creative Center's Artist Training

The fulfillment of The Creative Center's goal of more artists in more hospitals making art with more people depends on the quality of our artists' training programs and the number of artists who can be trained.

Locally, The Creative Center Artists-In-Residence are trained individually in response to the development of a new hospital or hospice position. These artists are drawn from applicants whose previous interviews suggest a good "fit" between the artist, the healthcare setting and The Center. Upon completion of the initial training and three day-long internships, the artists become part of our extensive program of supervision, retraining and creative enrichment.

National AIR Training

In response to requests for artist (AIR) training in healthcare settings from artists and hospital personnel outside the New York area, The Center initiated a National AIR Training Program for artists from other states and countries who meet in small groups in New York for a five-day intensified Artist-In-Residence training course. These artists return to their hometowns to use the training in a multiplicity of creative ways. Our on-line resources and personal availability provide on-going support to all our artists.

New York Area Creative Center (CC) Training Model

In order to give all the New York area artists the most comprehensive training for our AIR Program in hospitals and hospices, The Center has developed a professional training team that includes:

- The director of The CC Artist-In-Residence Program.
- CC Artists-In-Residence who have worked in healthcare settings for at least one year.
- Hospital administrators, ethicists and disease control specialists.
- Physicians, nurses and social workers.
- Artists and educators from museums, multi-media art studios and experiential workshops.

An artist's internship with Creative Center AIRs in healthcare settings is the core of The Center's training. *We believe that we all learn best by experiencing the concepts that are presented, and that we all contribute to each other's learning experiences.* As support for the internships, artists are given didactic and experiential training in the following areas:

- The human body.
- Cancer and other life-threatening illnesses.
- Medical protocol.
- Professional protocol.
- Patients, families, staff and their hospital experiences.
- Being a patient; being an artist.
- How to begin.
- Hospice and palliative care.
- Integrating your creativity into the hospital setting.
- Projects for working at the bedside.
- Developing resources and tactics for self-care.
- Evaluating the work.

As the artists learn about working in a healthcare setting, a foreign environment for most artists, all sorts of questions, conflicts and issues are addressed. Our training respects not only the artists' different learning styles and tempos, but also their individual levels of stress and their need for impromptu discussions and feedback. The Creative Center evaluates the artists' knowledge and comfort level with the requirements of their work as Artists-In-Residence, which enables us to further define individual training needs.

After the Training — Next Steps

After the artists complete their initial Creative Center training and fulfill the physical examination requirements of their assigned hospital, they take part in that hospital's orientation program for volunteers. The Artists-In-Residence, who typically work in their hospitals one to two days each week, are paid by The Center but are considered by the hospitals to be volunteers. This approach cuts through enormous institutional red tape, protects the artists under the insurance given to hospital volunteers, and provides a basic structure for integrating the AIRs into each healthcare setting.

The Director of our Artist-In-Residence Program and the hospital employee with whom we have negotiated the artist's residency decide on the *artist's hospital contact.* The new artist is introduced to the contact person, usually a nurse or a social worker, who in turn, introduces the artist to the staff on the floors where the artist will work. During the first week of residency, the artist is accompanied by a seasoned AIR who continues in the

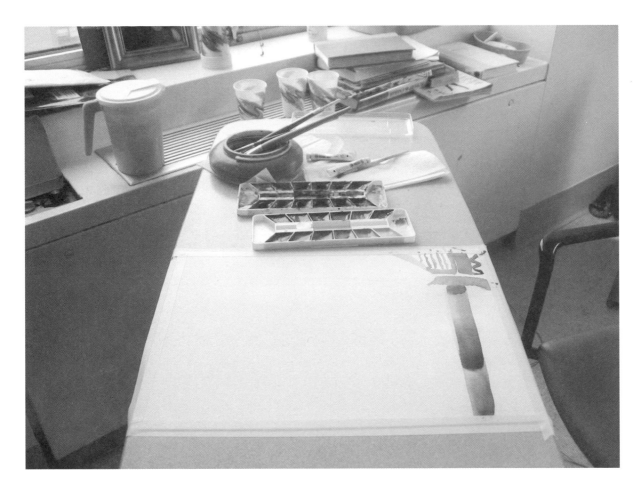

role of mentor and friend to the new Artist-In-Residence.

Encouragement, Support and Supervision

AIRs develop strong feelings for patients and staff alike, but at the end of the day, they often feel that it is a job that only another AIR can fully appreciate. Although AIRs can refer to The Center's ethical and professional guidelines, collection of first-day stories and samples of artists' logs, nothing is as meaningful as communicating directly with another AIR.

Every six weeks, all local AIRs attend an evening meeting at The Creative Center. The meeting begins with supper and includes administrative details, project demonstrations, educational presentations by invited guests, and open discussions about the beauty and the difficulty, the sadness and the joy, and the gifts, that are all a part of this work. In addition to these meetings, the director of the AIR program schedules site visits to each hospital and arranges individual supervisory time with each artist to review the content of the logs; discuss feedback from the hospital contact;

and offer suggestions and support for AIR experiences that range from the simple to the complex.

Artist Logs

All AIRs are responsible for written logs that describe each of their hospital workdays. The logs are turned in to The Center at the end of each month; they bear witness to the extraordinary work of the artists and to the hopeful and courageous spirit of patients, families and healthcare staff. (AIRs are instructed to change all names to ensure confidentiality.) Artists find that writing about their hospital experiences, about their patient and staff interactions, about artmaking, about miracles large and small, enables them to reflect upon and to integrate their work more fully.

As I look at my bag of materials I see a bag of possibilities and want to share and learn from the people I hope will want to work with me. I wonder, though, how people so ill will have the energy or the interest to work. I can only hope we can work on a project together that might lead to something else — perhaps a collaborative challenge to break patterns, expectations or fixed ideas.

Today was an exhausting, difficult day, and I felt terrible that I didn't have the power to do more for the people that I saw.

Louise said that as a result of her medicine her hands often shake, and because of that she doesn't think art making is in her future. I told her to embrace the uncontrollable nature of that, the unsteadiness and the movement in her line — that if she could let go of what she thinks a line is — and learn what her line is — she will open herself up to new possibilities. She thanked me and said I made her feel so much better, and that she will remind herself of that when she is feeling down. I am thinking perhaps these experiences and those that lie before me will influence my work and me in ways unimaginable.

I started to feel let down that so many people seemed to be too tired to be involved, or simply not interested, but I realized — one step at a time — after all this work isn't for me; it's for them and they will inevitably share with me what they are capable of. I can only be fortunate enough to be a part of the experience.

Working as an AIR

Creative Center artists often describe their work as hospital AIRs as one of the most important and meaningful experiences of their lives, and, regardless of the artistic medium, believe that these experiences inform their own artwork. *The Creative Center is committed to providing professional training and on-going support to all of our artists, whether based locally or nationally.*

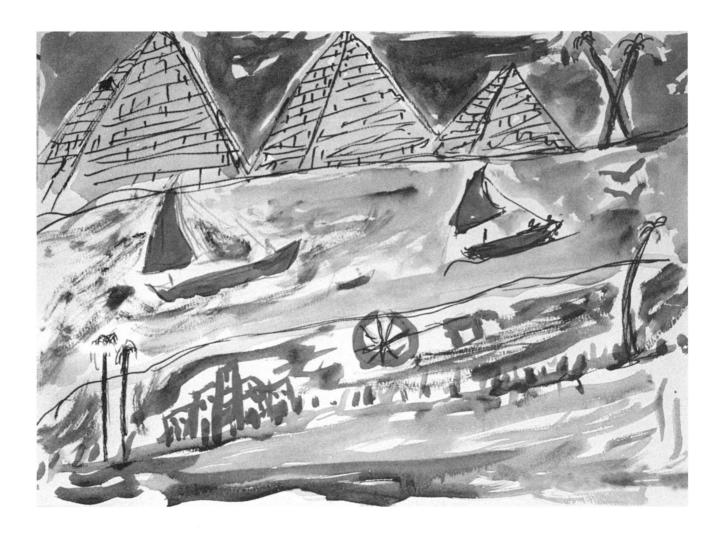

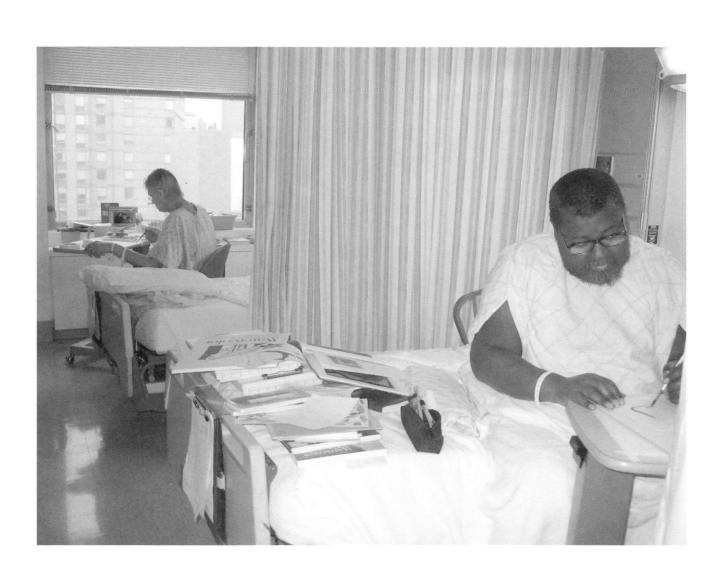

Reggie & Ken

February 22: *Reggie is a fifty-two-year-old, African-American man with lymphoma. His roommate, on the in-patient unit of the Infusion Suite, is Ken, who is sixty-three, Caucasian and also has cancer. Although I originally stopped in to see Reggie, both wanted to paint. Reggie said he'd done some art before. "I live in an SRO [single-room occupancy, low-income housing] and a nice lady comes to help us do art. I made some dinosaurs and other animals, then I didn't do it, then I did it again. It helps me with my self-esteem." Ken, a divorce and bankruptcy lawyer and amateur photographer, added, "I was just saying to a nurse this morning that I've been here so long I'm beginning to get antsy and was wishing there was something for me to do. Now here is an artist." Two people sharing a hospital room can exist very separately, relating little, as Reggie and Ken had — until art transformed the clinical setting into an art studio.*

While I was setting up, Reggie looked through a collection of reproductions of paintings and photographs to "wake up his creative juices." Ken paged through a book of abstract paintings that he liked. Each man received a 11" x 15" watercolor paper taped to a board, a set of paints, a container with water, two brushes (one large, one small), a small practice paper and paper towels. I stood in front of their beds and gave what I call my "three-minute watercolor lesson." Ken began first. It took Reggie a little longer to feel at ease. Just when he did, a nurse came by to say it was time for a test. Reggie was disappointed, as was I. I agreed to leave some art materials for both of them to use later.

As Ken worked, he talked about his children. "I waited a long time to get married and have children. They're twelve and fourteen. My ex-wife has been great since my illness; she knows how much the children love me." He said he'd always wanted to build a model boat or try painting, but never had. And he remembered Jackson Pollock, "What I'm doing reminds me of his paintings — did you see the movie? Trying this, I understand those paintings better." As he talked, he painted.

March 1: *"Oh, you should see the paintings Ken and his sister did! They're hanging in his room."* This was the excited greeting I received from the head nurse upon my arrival. I was anxious to see the paintings. Having had minor surgery, Ken was not up to painting, saying apologetically, *"I'm sorry I don't have more art questions."* I replied, *"Don't worry. It's a pleasure just to see you."* Words that made him say, *"That's sweet."*

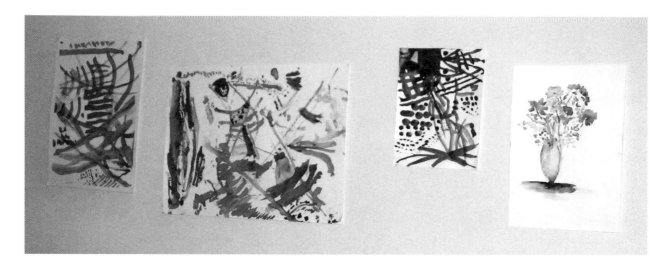

March 8: *Two weeks ago I met two very different men, who by now have been roommates for a month. The first week we worked together, Ken made two paintings. Returning the next week I wasn't able to work with Reggie, but saw three paintings Ken and his sister Suzanne had done. Today, Reggie was in the room alone, a large and gentle, meticulous man. He showed me a crayon painting he'd completed — a group of simple images that display his fondness for animals, imaginative spirit and ability to create complex colors with only a few crayons. "Sometimes it's hard for me to focus and get my creativity going," Reggie remarked. "I'll do an abstract," he declared, sketching forms onto his watercolor paper. A nurse interrupted, asking for a urine sample. I excused myself and went to the patient lounge to write some notes. My presence awakened a man resting on the couch. It was Ken who explained that he didn't sleep well at night, "I sleep best in here. I'm glad you found me. I would have been disappointed if I had missed you."*

"I'm ready," Reggie called out as Ken and I entered the room. Ken showed me the three fine brushes and two tubes of watercolors his sister had sent him.

I marveled at the art he'd done during the week. As the two worked, I went back and forth between them, offering encouraging comments or creative suggestions as needed. After Ken painted some linear shapes, he wasn't sure where to go with his painting. Looking out the window, he said, "Look at the swirling snow." "Why don't you get that motion into your painting?" I suggested. Meanwhile, Reggie worked meticulously on a small, complex painting. His decisions as to how and where to sign his name and place his brushstrokes were executed with delicacy and assurance. Both men were pleased with the paintings they made during our session, and both agreed they wanted to do more. After hanging the recently created works, I gave the residents of the newly-christened "Artists-at-Work" studio and gallery (formerly only a hospital room) the art supplies necessary to continue with the art making. Ken and Reggie's gallery was good for the nurses and aides too, giving the staff something to be proud of and lifting their spirits.

March 17: *Today, one month after I met them, Ken and Reggie are still in the hospital and both have become dedicated painters — their room transformed into a gallery. They had been roommates and diligent artists until the previous night when Ken had been moved to the Critical Care Unit (CCU). As I greeted Reggie and he was telling me about the painting he'd made during the week, I noticed that Ken's paintings were still on the walls. I instinctively gathered them for safekeeping, surprised at the intensity of my feelings. Later after my third attempt to see Ken in the CCU, I found his ex-wife and sister and gave them his work. "He was so happy painting. It meant so much to him," they told me.*

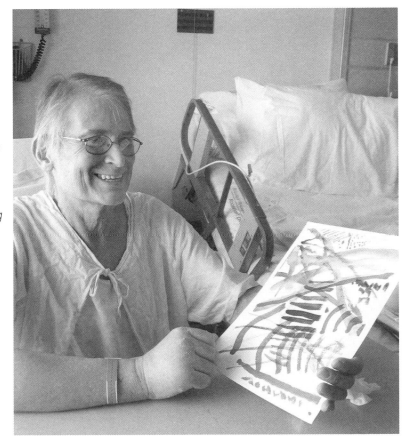

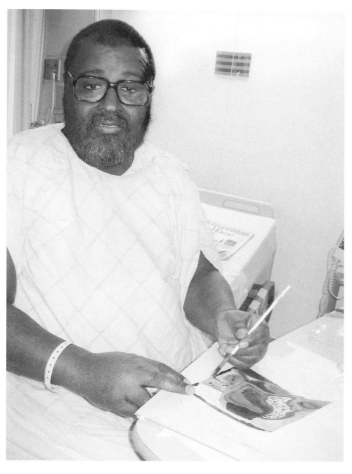

I took pictures of Reggie and his new painting. He was proud of his achievements and glad to have a visual record of his accomplishment.

March 22: *"How's Ken?"* was the first question I asked upon my arrival. I learned that he was still in the CCU and not doing well. Continuing to work with Reggie filled some of my sadness about Ken, but it added to it, too. Reggie was anxious to show me his three new pieces. I rearranged his paintings on the wall in front of his bed, including his new ones and the photos of him working. This display had a positive effect on all who saw it. Comments about his work made Reggie happy and proud; he clearly loves painting.

March 29: Today I learned that Ken had died. I first met him five weeks ago, and within the first moments of working with him, I knew he might die soon. Although he intermittently seemed disoriented and clearly had physical problems, his gentle spirit and eagerness to paint never waned. Ken's ability to take each moment as it happened had a mesmerizing affect on me, not to mention his natural ability to paint abstractly. On a printout of photographs I took of him working that I hung amidst his paintings, I wrote *"Ken has a natural affinity for the abstract."* This made Ken laugh; his pleasure made me laugh, too. There was something about Ken's manner that made it easy to be with him, even while it was painful to see him lose the direction of his thoughts and actions, and to observe his gout-bloated hands and legs. *"Goodbye, Ken. I'm so glad I met you."*

I said a different goodbye to Reggie, the meticulous man of many paintings. He went home last Friday; I'd thought I would get to work with him at least one more time. As I will miss Ken, I will miss Reggie, too, although I can imagine Reggie making artwork in future days…painting and drawing.

Working in the Unique Culture of a Healthcare Institution

Hospitals are characterized by their own peculiar institutional culture — values, philosophies and ideologies; formal and informal organizational structures; protocols, rules and regulations. The business of restoring health and saving lives is complicated. Creating a balance between financial solvency and providing up-to-date medical care to all who need it is challenging.

Mission, Vision and Values

Like most corporate entities, each healthcare institution has developed its own mission, vision and values statements to guide its plans and actions. Regardless of the size or affiliation of the institution, these principles are remarkably similar. **Mission statements** proclaim a striving for excellence in medical services with a sincere commitment to patient care. **Vision statements** see the institution as THE leader in medical expertise in its geographical service area.

Most **value statements** contain some variation on the following:

- Our patients receive excellent care, delivered with compassion.
- Each of our employees and volunteers is a valued member of the team.
- We respect the integrity and diversity of every person.
- We are good stewards of our resources, now and for the future.
- We strive to be a responsible, contributing member of our community.

Many faith-based institutions and some others have an additional value: honoring the health of the whole person — body, mind and spirit.

When artists come to work at a particular healthcare institution, they are joining an established culture. Everything runs cautiously and carefully and may feel unbearably slow to an artist who is used to acting quickly and independently. Decisions come from the top down and, currently, professionals — the administration and physicians — direct patient care. Increasingly, patients are seeking alternative and additional sources of healing beyond traditional allopathic medicine. Healthcare institutions have responded by offering more alternative and complementary options, such as Artists-In-Residence. Future trends indicate that healthcare will become increasingly patient driven and concerned with treating the whole person.

When I first arrived I met with Janet, the social worker. She wanted to chat and see how things were going and suggest who I might stop to work with. She said there were many patients who had contagious illnesses or were just too ill to be bothered. So I listened and stayed away from those people. I wonder if the nurses can see them, then why can't I? I would wear the necessary protection. I just sometimes think, those are the people who might be most in need of some artwork and extra attention.

The Facility and the People Within

Hospitals thrive on organization and are continually organizing. Physically they are set up in units or floors, each one specializing in the care of a particular medical diagnosis. Some designations include: Oncology, Labor and Delivery, Rehabilitation, Bone Marrow Transplant, Pediatrics, Surgery, Intensive Care. Generally the larger the institution, the more specialized the unit can be and the more of them there are. The physicians and nurses who work on each unit often have earned certification in that specialty.

A staff hierarchy exists at most institutions — beginning with the **physicians** who may be MDs or DOs (doctor of osteopathic medicine, a degree with training very similar to the MD). Physicians generally are not hospital employees and do not have offices at the hospital; they appear periodically to make rounds on their patients. They are responsible for all care decisions. **Social workers** provide patients and families with psychosocial support needed to cope with hospitalization and illness. **Nurses** provide direct, bedside patient care and carry out medical regimens (they are the largest group of healthcare workers in the US with most of them working in hospitals). **Registered nurses (RNs)** and **certified nurse practitioners (CNPs)** have graduated from accredited schools of nursing and are licensed to practice by a state authority. CNPs have more education, and so more responsibility in patient care. **Licensed practical nurses (LPNs or licensed vocational nurses, LVNs,** in some parts of the country) have less education, responsibility and fewer skills. **Orderlies** and **nurses aides** take orders from RNs and LPNs and help with patient basic care.

Other members the healthcare team may include are a chaplain, child life specialist and a variety of therapists. The **chaplain** makes daily rounds and is available around-the-clock to provide pastoral care, crisis intervention and spiritual support for patients, family and staff. **Child life specialists** are guided by the philosophy of "family-centered care." They supervise play as therapy or diversion; prepare children for and assist them during medical tests and procedures; and support families during hospitalization or challenging events. Types of **therapists** include: creative arts (including art, music, dance/movement, drama, poetry, psychodrama, biblio, photo and expressive arts), occupational and recreational. The work of these people differs from that of an AIR. Therapists have completed certified training and have learned to treat the patient with a particular outcome in mind — they assess needs and strengths, identify specific goals, develop a program with specific activities, and evaluate the program's effectiveness.

As the meeting continued, it dawned on me that I didn't know what recreational therapists do with patients, so I asked. After a long pause, Rochelle took up the gauntlet and explained how, as a recreational therapist, she spent time with a patient assessing their cognitive and physical abilities and mood, and then making a treatment plan. The plan includes sensory stimulation through color, sound, smell and touch awareness. The director then commented that the goal of the Therapeutic Recreation team is to treat symptoms of the patients (pain, shortness of breath, anxiety, depression, isolation) and this is what is kept in mind as materials are brought to people. This information helped me understand how my approach to the creative process as an Artist-In-Residence is continuous with and different from the methods of recreational therapists.

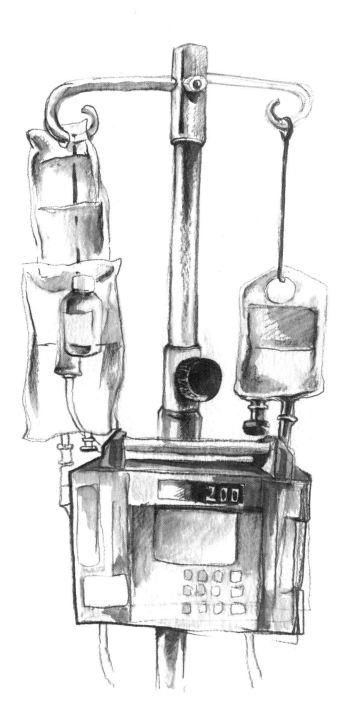

In a teaching hospital, another multi-faceted layer is added — **physicians-in-training: fellows, residents, interns** and **students.** Fellows fall just below physicians in status and are MDs or DOs who have completed medical school, internship, residency (specialty training) and are now studying a sub-specialty. Sub-specialty study can last anywhere from one to five or six years after a residency of two to five years. Not every physician is required to do an internship, the year between medical school and residency. During the third and fourth years of medical school, students spend time in different clinical rotations on the hospital's units. A family or internal medicine physician has typically trained for seven years after college; an interventional cardiologist, eleven.

On the floors, a **nurse manager** or **charge nurse** is responsible for administering one or more units. This individual works the regular hours of a normal business week. Floor nurses and aides work in shifts as the hospital must be staffed 24/7. Some hospitals work three 8-hour shifts daily, others have moved to 12-hour shifts/36 hour weeks. Other staff the AIR may interact with are **food service, environmental services (janitorial/housekeeping), administration/clerical** and **facilities/construction.**

By the time I fill my cart with supplies and wheel it towards the bone marrow transplant unit, it is just after noon. I've learned about the hospital's paging system through a series of initially fruitless attempts to page the facilities manager for the 10th floor (who has the keys to our storage locker); again found my way through the labyrinthian basement back to the locksmith's shop in the Security Office (a duplicate key needed to be picked up); learned about the automated Sabbath elevator which stops on every floor (supposedly after 4 on Fridays but apparently all day today); and have gotten my first sense of the inner workings of a hospital. I'm amazed at the web of individuals involved in its smooth functioning: the cleaning staff with their carts loaded with mops and clear buckets filled with pink and green and yellow disinfecting fluid; the receptionists at the nurses' stations in each unit who announce, to the shifting crowd of doctors, nurses, and technical staff, the name of the paged-person returning their call; the teams of doctors, nurses and social workers who periodically gather outside patients' rooms for what look like strategy sessions, pep talks or football huddles; and many others. It's fascinating to me. The huge windows, filled with a dramatic view from on high of the East River, Roosevelt Island and the FDR, makes all of the bustling activity seem almost mythically significant.

Becoming Part of the Patient Care Team

The culture of healthcare is not the same as the one that surrounds art. Just as the artist probably knows little about patient care and the practice of medicine, so those who are clinically based may have limited familiarity with an Artist-In-Residence, what you do and why. Many have never thought about having the arts be a part of healthcare. Your job as an AIR will include educating and working with the healthcare staff. You may offer a creative experience — a lunchtime artmaking workshop in the nurses' lounge, an invitation to an opening or an exhibition. Leave a small gift to brighten their environment: a handmade card, an art reproduction or an art calendar. While they are often overworked and very busy, they will appreciate your efforts and look forward to your presence.

Staff may be initially concerned with how much extra work artmaking will mean for them. An effective AIR is friendly with all of the staff encountered on the unit. Respect their space; you are coming into their culture. They are the patient care team of which you will be come a valued member. Be willing to do anything possible to make their jobs easier. On that team, nurses and social workers are generally an artist's most important allies. As the ones most directly responsible for patient care, they can make suggestions about which patients to visit and answer all kinds of questions knowledgeably.

After some further administrative business, I accompanied Betty (Director of Therapeutic Recreation) to an interdisciplinary team meeting. These meetings are attended by some or all of the following: doctor, nurse, nutritionist, pharmacist, discharge planner, social worker, recreational therapist, music therapist, artist. Betty introduced me to these people (and everyone else I met that day) with these words: "This is Lilly Brown. She is a professional artist who will be working at the bedside with patients." This lovely and accurate description of my purpose puts me in a state of happy amazement. I can hardly believe that they have had the insight to include the opportunity to make art as part of their mission of "non-abandonment" for patients and those who love them. After the meeting, Betty and I proceeded to each floor and each unit (two per floor), where I was introduced to doctors, nurses, social workers — people who need to know why I am there so they can refer patients they think would benefit from this service. Some were surprised, but everyone was welcoming.

The nurses seem to be paying more attention. They speak longer and seem to wait for responses. They listen to my replies and want to engage in conversation. They have, on different occasions, told me how important the work I do is. If I'm working in a room, they seem to linger a while as they walk past; they comment on the process — making a joke or taking time to walk around the bed to see what the patient is doing. It's really working here. I got the nurses on board. I don't know who or how, but they are all on a team — and, hey, I'm on that team, too! It's a great feeling. I look forward to walking the halls, and I don't mind the down time when I just sit and think about the rejections. They even joke with me as I sit by the window, never prodding me but respecting the difficulty of getting a taker. Sometimes they offer a room number or two. "Try Room 45. She might be interested." Sometimes when I walk into Room 45, I can't believe they thought it was a possibility, and sometimes they are right, so right about who they think will work. It's really, really good these days.

AIRs work in a hospital because they have something unique to offer not only patients and families, but everyone on staff. *An AIR can model imaginative thinking within the highly structured environment of healthcare; offer passion for the arts in an unlikely place; inspire individuals to think of themselves and their situations in creative ways.*

Respecting Protocols and Boundaries

In a healthcare institution, establishing and respecting boundaries becomes particularly important in order to protect the health of the patient, family, staff and volunteers. From infection prevention to protecting confidentiality, the hospital has rules and regulations that are *not* open to creative interpretation.

Hospital protocols

Hospitals have many "protocols" — sets of conditions everyone is to follow under specific circumstances. Protocols exist for infection control, treatments of different diseases and conditions, hand washing, reporting errors, confidentiality and much more. *A hospital's specific protocols are not to be interpreted creatively, but followed exactly.* Each hospital site will teach the AIR their particular regulations and requirements during the AIR's orientation process.

Hospitals have particular protocols for preventing the spread of infection. A serious, on-going concern is *nosocomial infections,* a type of infection a patient can acquire just from being in the hospital. AIRs should take seriously, and follow rigorously, all prevention protocols in order to safeguard the health of their patients as well as their own.

- Wash hands often and thoroughly.
- Wear a gown or mask.
- Disinfect art supplies between patients.
- Do whatever is required to minimize the spread of infection.

HIPAA, a federal law — the Health Insurance Portability and Accountability Act of 1996 — requires a patient's permission to disclose or use any medical information. This law is to ensure patient privacy and confidentiality; hospitals take it very seriously, although the AIR may hear complaints or jokes about the added forms or extra work involved.

Medical protocols

The Creative Center has developed these basic medical protocols that all AIRs should observe:

1. Do not go to the hospital if you are ill.

2. The instinct to touch another person as an expression of compassion is integral to our humanity. However,

in the hospital setting it is imperative that the patient's attending nurse or physician approves all physical contact before it is initiated. The exception is holding the patient's hand, but it is important to ask the patient first.

3. Wash your hands before and after working with each patient *(see box, upper right)*.

4. Do not touch the patient's medical equipment; it is to be handled by staff members only.

5. Use only the staff bathrooms.

6. Use only safe, non-toxic art materials.

7. Patients who are in isolation have special protocols *(see box, lower right)* that must be observed in order to protect the patient and yourself. Patients undergoing stem cell and bone marrow transplants, or who have any condition that severely impairs the immune system, are at a high risk of developing life-threatening infections.

8. Report your patient's suicidal thoughts and/or preparations to their nurse or social worker.

9. Report (immediately!) sudden changes in your patient's physical and mental state — anything requiring medical assistance including loss of consciousness, hallucinations, intense pain that has become unmanageable, or breathing problems — i.e. choking.

- Press the nurse call button.
- Go for help.
- Do not touch the patient.

PROPER TECHNIQUE FOR HAND WASHING

Wash your hands properly to kill germs and prevent infection:

1. Use warm running water.

2. Lather hands well with liquid soap, if available, and scrub with vigor for as long as it takes to sing "Happy Birthday."

3. Pay special attention to nails, between fingers and around rings. (Rings can trap germs; it's better to remove them while working in the hospital.)

4. Rinse thoroughly.

5. Dry with paper towel. (Avoid using a cloth towel that can transmit germs back to your clean hands.)

6. Put the paper towel over your hand to turn off the water tap.

ISOLATION PROTOCOLS

Before entering the isolation patient's room:

1. Ask the nurse if the patient can receive visitors.

2. If the patient can receive visitors, ask the nurse what safety measures you need to follow.

3. Wash hands and put on necessary protective coverings.

When you are with the patient in the isolation room:

1. Do not touch the patient.

2. *Use art materials purchased for that patient only; isolation patients cannot share materials.*

Today I shadowed Ben at his hospital. We primarily visited patients on the bone marrow transplant unit, confined to private rooms. Throughout the day I learned the protocols for working with immune-compromised patients — everything from dressing gowns to constantly washing our hands. I truly expected this but I didn't expect to have such a strong sense of how isolating this type of hospitalization can be. The rooms have double doors with a washing area in between so there is really no contact until a person "suits up," washes up and comes in to the second doorway. I had no idea that I would spend so much time dressing and undressing, making laundry of those yellow precautionary gowns! The hospital has outfitted these rooms with computers and exercise bikes and they are spacious, but somehow none of it seemed to make up for that double-doored separation from the rest of the world.

Respecting the patient's boundaries

When a person becomes hospitalized, he surrenders, by necessity, much of his personal privacy and control. Offering the hospitalized patient the luxury of choice may be one of the most important aspects of the AIR's work. While you are committed to artmaking, you should remain flexible and responsive — the value of your interchange with patients rests on respecting their remaining boundaries.

1. *Respect the patient's privacy.* Make your presence known by knocking and asking permission to enter the room.
2. *Respect the patient's space.* Stay off the bed; sit in a chair, being sure to allow the staff easy access to the patient.

3. *Refrain from wearing perfume or after-shave.* Patients may have allergies or difficulty breathing.
4. *Wires, IVs, machines, food or beverage, help to the bathroom, etc. are off-limits to the AIR.* If a patient needs assistance with anything medical, notify the nurse. If the patient says or does anything worrisome, notify the social worker or nurse.
5. *It's all about being with the patients.* Let them talk; be curious about their lives and ask questions; listen and respond. They and their families are your top priority.
6. *The AIR's area of expertise is artmaking.* Offering advice or suggestions about other subjects is inappropriate.
7. *If staff arrives, ask them if they would like you to leave the room*

while they treat the patient. Find out when you may return, either to continue working with the patient or to clean up. Most interruptions are brief.

8. *Maintain the confidentiality* of what is seen and heard at all times; it's not only appropriate and respectful, but it's the law (HIPAA). You may discuss patient information only in conference with other staff and with your supervisor or contact person.

Today she didn't want to work — she was weak and felt ill. But she wanted to talk. I sat down and she just talked and slowly I got her to play with some materials. She thanked me saying, sometimes you just don't know what you need. She let me know it relaxed her and took her mind off herself. She said art is like its own medicine.

She told me about her life — her kids — one on parole, one dropped out of high school, another who gets jumped just walking to school.

Left with nothing, and so ill, and just wanting to do anything to help her children…I wonder…what is the miracle that could help her?

As things got heavier and I felt myself biting my tongue and wishing so much to be able to do something more — to have more art materials to lay in front of her…I thought of leaving…

But I realized she needed to talk — to let it all out. I listened and helped her write a letter to her children.

Respecting your own boundaries

Working with patients can become frustrating, sad, emotional…and overwhelming. It's important to take care of yourself so you can continue to be of service, physically, emotionally and artistically to patients. There are no rules about self-care other than it should help you feel restored, comforted or relaxed.

1. *Be aware of overload* and stop before it's reached. When you're feeling like it's too much, remove yourself from the scene. Get a cup of coffee; take a walk.

2. *Establish a contact person* on the unit; communicate with that person frequently (once a week). If you are unable to come to work, notify your contact person and your supervisor.

3. *Develop personal tools* to help you keep your balance; talk to other AIRs; write in your log.

4. *Dress comfortably;* layers of clothes will help you be prepared for hospital temperatures that often vary. AIRs have reported that patients respond positively to colorful outfits — if this suits your personality and wardrobe, do it!

5. *Keep personal contact information personal.* If a patient wants a way to reach you, give the workplace telephone number.

6. *AIRs do not visit patients outside the hospital.* If someone asks, be prepared to suggest sources for art supplies and other artmaking opportunities in your community.

I find it very therapeutic if I go ice-skating before going to work in the hospital; all that cold fresh air, exercise and good music clears my head, and relaxes my body.

The morning was over and it was time for my break. The morning flew by — I'm in fast forward today. I have to remember to slow down sometimes. I tend to let the energy carry me but I think I need to pay more attention to what I am doing, as I am doing it.

She said it was nice to just be able to talk to someone like when she used to work and have conversations with her co-workers. When it was time for me to go, she asked (out of the blue), "Do you get depressed being here?" I asked what she meant and she asked if being around so many sick people was depressing. I said that no, I really enjoyed working together as we had today and looked forward to seeing her Tuesday. She seemed satisfied and smiled saying, "Well then, we have plenty to do," and said goodbye.

The AIR, a Valuable Addition to the Healthcare Culture

This chapter has been about navigating that particular, peculiar culture which exists in a healthcare institution. An artist can add to the environment by modeling creativity and imagination, but *to be effective, the AIR must follow the institution's written (and unwritten) rules and protocols, and respect everyone's boundaries.* By gaining the trust of the patients, families and staff, the artist will become a model of creative expression and a valued member of the healthcare team.

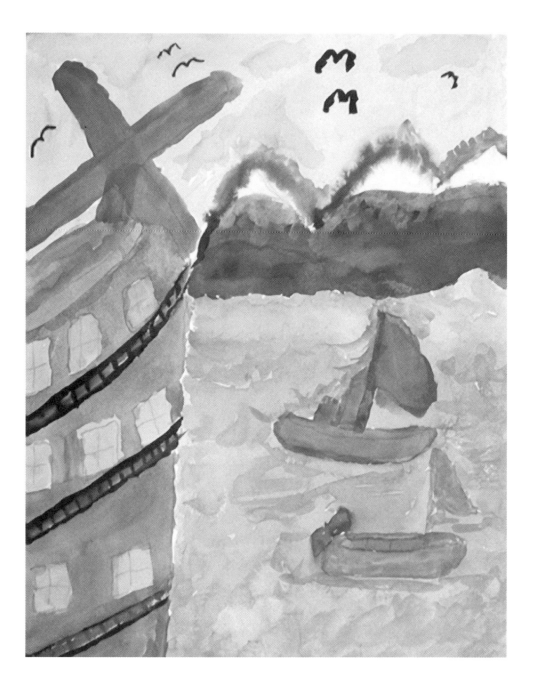

He needed to lie flat for a while as his legs were bothering him but he said he hoped to paint later on. So I covered the paints and checked in with a care technician who agreed to help clean up later. Before saying goodbye he thanked me again and then talked a bit more about his plans to make a castle and a cruise ship. It's been great to see Terry use the art to express himself, to relate to the staff (who adore his sculptures and bring others in to see them) and to create some respite from his constant pain. He often thanks me but I've truly enjoyed creating artwork and talking with him.

Working with Patients

It was a simple visit. A bit of positive encouragement, slight technical help and, most importantly, some quiet company. It's during these times that I realize how powerful the work of The Creative Center is and, how important my work is as an Artist-In-Residence. I invite people to be creative, to join me in something productive that may not have anything to do with being in the hospital or dying, that focuses on their strengths rather than on their physical challenges. I am not a medical practitioner, caring family member or volunteer; I come to them as an artist, bringing my skills, enthusiasm and flexibility. Even people who aren't that interested in artmaking often want to talk, and sometimes there is a palpable relief at being able to just be with someone who doesn't need them to be a "good" patient or family member. I am honored to be with these ordinary yet amazing individuals, and so very grateful to have this precious opportunity to be part of this special work.

Working with all patients can be intimate, intense, difficult and, frequently, thrilling. *As an AIR, your ability to come up with creative approaches to a myriad of bedside situations will be well tested.* Responding creatively to each patient's individuality and abilities is at the heart of working as an artist in a hospital.

Scenario — An AIR's Visit

And in you walk — after knocking and hearing someone say — "Come in." Your response might be, "Hello, I am an Artist-In-Residence on this floor; my name is Sarah Smith. I am here to make art with you." The patient, thunderstruck at your introduction, may reply, "An artist — in a hospital?"

As the scene unfolds, take a deep breath and make a quick assessment of what you see, hear and smell; perhaps the most important clue to this assessment is what you immediately feel. A room full of light, color and family members will impart a very different feeling from one in which the shades are drawn and the patient is alone. Depending on multiple factors, including the artist's personality, energy level and overall arts in healthcare experience, the initial dialog with the patient may focus on small talk, on the patient's physical status or on the possibilities of making art.

The patient may say, "Oh, I haven't made art since the fourth grade." Or, "I can't draw a straight line." Or, "I am too — sick, tired, anxious, in pain — to make any art." An artist could respond, "What do you like to do?" or ask about a picture, flowers or family photographs in the room.

Typically, if a conversation gets rolling, artmaking can be reintroduced.

One AIR coaxed a patient, who looked too tired and weak to draw, into playing with clay — making beads for a necklace and a small dog. Another AIR brought in old articles about life on the East River to a man who had been a tugboat captain; the patient was drawn into painting endless studies of tugboats because he wanted to make sure the AIR understood what the boats were like in his day. Conversations often lead to unusual ways of incorporating art into the patient's hospital life.

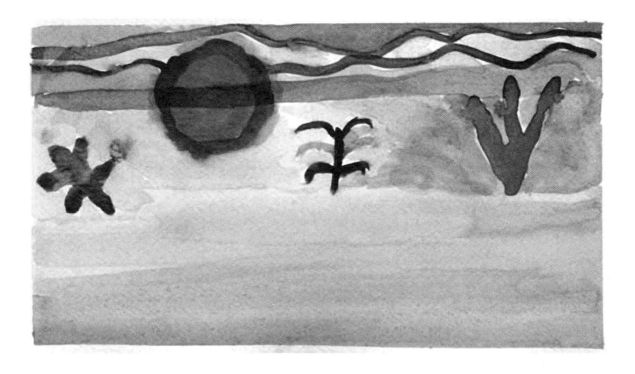

Mary engaged me in a long conversation today, asking with a wink if creative conversation counted as art. She told me about her yearly trips to the beach with her family, how she could count her life like rings on a tree by those summers at the beach. Her conversations are paintings — scenes from her life, ideas from a lifetime working as a nurse and living in her community, opinions that are steadfast, coupled with questions and wonderings that are philosophical. She creates a universe with her conversation, pulling in the nurses and housekeeping staff to talk, always running down that beach with a new kite of ideas in the air based on a small tidbit heard in passing.

Regardless of how enticing your offer is to make art, some patients will be too ill, tired, anxious, in too much pain or just resistant to make art themselves. You can offer various ways of working together on an art project, or let the patient art-direct your efforts. Artists often bring art books, catalogs or magazines to stimulate patients' interest in art. Looking at art publications together often leads to making art or to a conversation in which patients share stories that are remembered because of the time you are able to spend with them.

Today I worked with Barbara, a woman in her seventies; on her wall was an enormous collage comprised of her extended family. I asked if she made it and she said that her grandson did and added that she was incapable of doing any such thing, that she hadn't an artistic bone in her body.

I suggested she make a little collage for her grandson as a gesture of appreciation. I showed her an auction catalog of Impressionist paintings and assured her that with such beautiful images it would be impossible to make a bad collage. She declined. I started to cut up the catalog and assemble some pieces; she made suggestions. She told me about tapestries she had seen in Germany, and suggested I create a scene that would tell a story as the tapestry makers had done. But she would not take the scissors. She only wanted to direct.

I started to deliberately misunderstand her instructions; she became increasingly irritated by my apparent incompetence and finally took the materials out of my hands. She worked adamantly, showing me what she wanted. A half hour passed without her looking up while she constructed a beautiful single panel. Then she explained the narrative to me. Finally she said, "See?! That's what I was saying." She added she had no intention of sending it to her grandson.

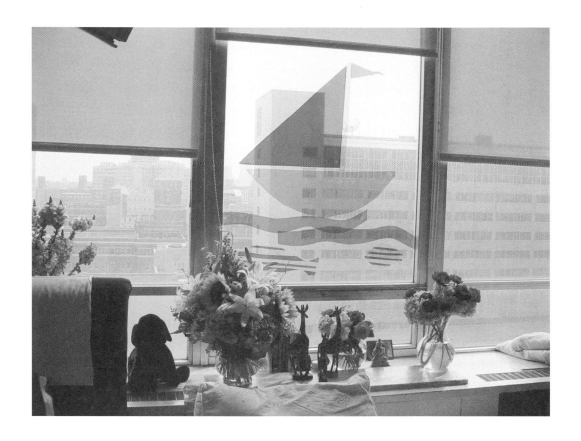

I got Ramon's handsome grandson started with colored gels, tape and scissors and he worked the rest of the day and into the early hours of the evening cutting out the translucent colored shapes for the window in the room his grandfather shared with a man who, curled in a fetal position, was moaning softly about his pain. Ramon was kind to the roommate, asking him what he would like to have on the window. At first the roommate, who really was in a lot of pain, didn't care. Before long, however, the pain and the not caring turned to rapt attention as he watched what was taking place on the window. After a time he sat up on the side of his bed gazing at Ramon, and smiling. Ramon cut palm trees and islands, landscapes, boats and skies with clouds and a sun. He wanted to be frugal with my supplies, so he cut many tiny pieces and wove them into a beautiful Dominican Republic world, a world far away from the pain enclosed by the gray walls of the hospital.

The Importance of Offering Choices

Choice is an important part of how the AIR presents creative experiences. In addition to giving a patient the choice of whether or not to work with you and who will do the work, The Creative Center employs AIRs, conversant in a variety of art modalities, who offer patients a range of art projects that use a variety of art materials. Our artists are continually exchanging ideas, tips and insights into making art with patients at the bedsides and in clinic settings.

Almost any artistic medium can be brought into a healthcare setting — visual art, music, drama, poetry, performance, etc. The Creative Center has received grants that have funded the work of writers and dancers as AIRs, further extending the choices we offer to patients and their families.

Dancers and Writers as AIRs

Dance, sometimes referred to as "movement," is one of the more unusual art forms a hospital can integrate. The Center's Dancer-In-Residence describes her work:

The biggest challenge as a dancing AIR is to convince both patients and staff that dancing is a great way to overcome the physical and mental frustration of lying in bed all day — even if you are still in bed when you dance. I create a space for patients to have an experience of themselves other than their illness. I find out what their favorite kind of music is, pop a CD into my portable player, and while we talk, I start to move to the music, leading them gently into a dance with me. For a moment they can be themselves on the dance floor again or at a jazz concert, or just goofing around to the radio.

If the patient cannot really move very much, we try to feel the beat of the music with either our fingers or our toes; if they have the energy, we imagine movements. I sometimes tell them that what they cannot do, I can do for them at their direction. And, when they don't have the words, my experience as a dancer can give them all sorts of choices.

If we agree to three choices in a row, we have a sequence of movements — a phrase of dance. Now we can make a dance. We dance together; we dance alone; I dance for you. The dance is amazing because as intricate as it is, we have never left our seats. It is all the more wonderful because something has not been done to you — something has come out of you.

Writing with patients in the hospital is more common. Poetry, memoir and journaling are some of the ways in which writers engage patients in reflection and self-expression.

For the medical staff, it is often enough to receive a mono-word answer, sometimes even a monosyllable from their patients. It becomes enough for the patient too. But it's not enough for me. I prodded and stalled and waited until there was some flow to Alice's voice, until she herself recognized it, until she owned her own voice and wanted to use it. It was then I proposed that we write. Alice untied the ribbon from the roll of blue paper that she had pulled from my carpetbag, and read what was written there: "Once again, tell me what it was like." That gave us a starting point.

When I went to see Nancy, she complained about the boredom and the routine of the hospital, so it was a good opportunity for me to produce pen and paper and offer them to her. She looked at the paper for a few moments and began to write. She wrote about children and about being around them a lot as a teacher; she wrote about how much she loves teaching, has always loved it from the very beginning, a few decades ago when she worked with kindergarteners. As she listed some of the children by name, discussed their antics, she even mentioned the clothing she wore back then: shoes with four-inch heels and short skirts, because longer skirts dragged on the floor. As she finished reading her piece there were tears in her eyes, but they weren't all tears of sadness. "I haven't thought about some of these kids in years," she said. "I'll bet some of them could do with someone thinking about them these days. And here I was sitting here believing that I had nothing left to think about."

When the Patient Says "No!"

Inevitably, there will be days when no one is well enough or interested enough to work with the AIR. It is difficult not to take the patients' refusals as rejections of what you are offering. It is even more difficult not to take their refusals personally. Consider, however, that you, the artist, may be the only person to whom patients have the power to say "no." Other healthcare staff tells the patient what to do and when to do it. There are very few opportunities for the patient to refuse or to make arbitrary decisions. *One of the most valuable aspects of offering artmaking in a hospital is the artist's ability to give the patient creative freedom of choice.* You are still doing your job — even if the patient says "no."

The goal of my work is artmaking, but I get confused about what this means. Artmaking is improvising, reading a situation, connecting with someone and creating a project with which I think they might feel comfortable. Frequently, when I enter a patient's room and initiate a conversation and they say, "No, no I'm not interested in making art," I will still have the sense that the patient doesn't quite want me to leave, so I stay and talk with them. Sometimes these conversations last a long time, and usually I reintroduce the idea of making art.

I started to feel let down that so many people seemed to be too tired to be involved, or simply not interested, but I realized — one step at a time — that after all, this work is not for me, it's for them, and they will inevitably share with me what they are capable of and what they desire. I can only be fortunate enough to be a part of that experience.

Keeping the Patient Your Main Focus

The ability to remain constantly and consistently in the moment with the patient is central to the work of an AIR. When you work with a patient, it is "all about" that patient — making him or her central to the creative experience. An AIR can bring fun and laughter, encouragement, support and validation to a patient's hospital experience. AIRs are there to draw out and interact with the whole patient by using every means at their disposal. With the patient's permission, some AIRs make art as well — both artist and patient drawing or painting. One AIR sketches patients' portraits as they work, giving them the finished artworks.

The Creative Center's AIR training underscores an artist's need to be flexible, adaptable and encouraging. Approaching work in this way enables both the patient and the AIR to feel good about their time together. An AIR's sensitivity allows him to interpret and respond to a patient's changeable moods, the inclusion of family members and the inconvenience of interruptions. Occasionally, a gentle persistence may be what patients need to distract them from their boredom, anxiety or pain.

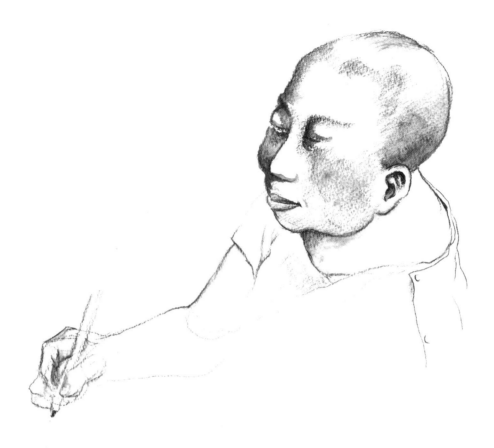

Hairless and depressed are two words that came to mind as Mike looked up at me, and said, "I'm in a funk; I can't do anything. My fingers don't work; the cancer has taken a lot from me." Instead of paying attention to his words, I began paying attention to his actions as he looked through the papers I had laid before him. I couldn't be sure, but he seemed interested in the watercolor papers, so I quickly opened both paints and water, and suggested he begin by trying out the colors. The surprising thing was that once Mike began, his attention was completely focused and his hands seemed to be working well. I was afraid to give many instructions or suggestions for fear of losing what appeared to be a thin thread of interest. But the more he worked the more focused he became. He later told me that he is a hairdresser, and that the two paintings he just made were the first he's done in thirty years.

Today I met with a nineteen-year-old girl with leukemia. After I introduced myself she politely declined my invitation to make art and turned away; her mother, who insisted I stay, decided to paint a still life with watercolors. As the mother began to paint, I asked her daughter about the lunch that she was ignoring. We looked at it together, trying to identify various parts of it. I suggested we design her fantasy lunch right there on her table. I covered the entire surface with white paper and gave her a box of colored pencils. It started out simply enough: burger, fries, diet Coke, but soon grew increasingly fantastic; more paper was patched over existing items; animals appeared — fish, crustaceans, flowers, elaborate pastries. Her mother continued to paint, as she furtively beamed at her daughter's energy. We worked irreverently, childishly; she was having a ball. She asked me if it was okay that she was doing this

instead of painting a still life. I told her that whatever made her feel better and wasn't illegal was permissible. When we were all done, she choked down her real lunch between bouts of laughter. Her mom's painting went up on the wall. The concocted lunch went into her mother's bag.

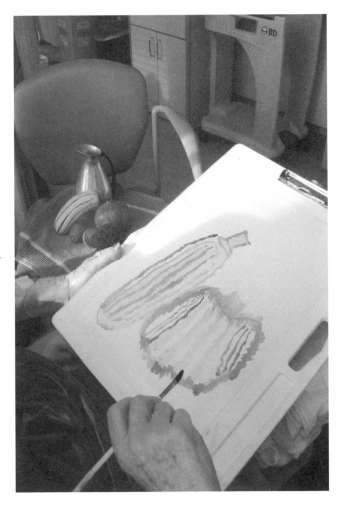

Denise decided to make a bracelet. I was surprised because when I first went in she looked miserable. Her roommate was in terrible pain, and said she couldn't bring herself to do anything; that the only sanity-saving thing for her has been the view of the river. If only that river knew how important it is in the life of so many people here. She was touched that she could choose all the pictures she wanted from those that I had for her room, and that she could see them when she woke up at night, which was quite often.

He was a hoot; I could have sworn he was from New Orleans, the Garden District by way of the French Quarter. He had all the nurses laughing and sauntering around him as he gave orders and compliments and criticisms, all with a deep Southern inflection in a voice that was obviously no stranger to the stage. He talked about life and love as he bellowed to the nurses, "Oh, come on girl, come on now, don't you look fine?" and they would prance around him. He was a King and a Queen at the same time, if you know what I mean. He was an opera singer, and heavens knows what else, but he was not given the gift of visual art. "No, darling," he said making it very clear to me. "Let's just try," I said.

He cleared his table and said something like, give it to me. He first drew a star like something you would see on top of a Christmas tree; I've seen this before, so I encouraged him. "What do you like? What do you love?" And he began to talk about this piano, how it sounds and how superior it was to a Steinway; he drew the candelabra on the top — "No, darling, not a candelabra, a luminaire." He drew the curtains around the piano and the Versaille floors; he drew all the panels that he explained were in the MET. And he talked about how he loved Germany and how they loved him back. He calmed down a bit, and we talked about talking to yourself and cancer and being in the world and in his piano room. He told me he was from a small town in upstate New York and he told me about the tumor on his neck and how you respond to that kind of news; I put the drawing of his piano room on his wall where he could plainly see it.

Without warning, Eileen surprised me by saying, you give me what I never had as a child — encouragement. "I never had a chance to be a child; I was an adult at seven." Wanting to continue to encourage her, I gave her a 4" x 6" drawing pad with the suggestion that she make the kind of drawings she had done at the hospital — images and words without censorship or judgment. "If you can't do that every day, do it when you can," I said, and left Eileen with the hope that she would make at least four drawings by the time she would come back to the hospital for her next treatment.

Working Long Term with Patients

In most cases, you will not know whether you will see the patient next week or perhaps ever again. This is often one of the most difficult aspects of the job as an Artist-In-Residence — *the tenuousness of relationships.*

Whether you will make art with a patient once or on many occasions is dictated in part by the type of facility or floor on which you work. Patients in bone marrow transplant units, in hospice care, or who come to an out-patient clinic for their radiation treatments may look forward to making art with you on a regular basis. Artists frequently devise on-going projects with which to involve and absorb these patients. Murals, poetry chapbooks and handwork are a few of the possibilities. Patients have the opportunity to develop their artmaking skills. Hospital rooms begin to look like art studios, drab clinics take on the appearance of quilting bees; and hospital staff and caregivers, who also must be there day-in and day-out, are happy to be surrounded by color and design. Patients often rearrange their clinic schedules so that they are there on "Artist Day."

Today I worked with a young man with no legs and a very sunny disposition. When I entered the room he asked if I was there with his legs. I apologized for being equipped only with art supplies. He said that he was struggling to write a poem on the occasion of his brother's wedding; making art might be just the thing. He had no experience, but handily put together a little collage on a sheet of cardstock that I had folded in half. It was a perfect card and needed only a word or two inside to be complete. He was amazed and proud; he felt like he just solved the whole enterprise of gift-giving. He positively loved doing it. We talked and worked and talked and worked some more; he was beaming. By the time I left, he had half-a-dozen outstanding cards for a multitude of upcoming occasions. I had a few of my own. "This is my new hobby; I'm not kidding!" he said ecstatically. I left him a small pile of catalogs, glue — the works. I suspect that someone somewhere is right now enjoying one of his gifts, saying something like, "I had no idea you could do this!" Neither did he.

It takes some getting used to, this business of not knowing if one will get to see a patient for a second or third time. I was looking forward to visiting several people from the previous week and all had been discharged, or had gone home. My happiness for the fact that they had moved on was wrapped up with a sense of unfinished business, of not doing more when I had the opportunity. On the other hand, I was delighted to see a patient who had just been re-admitted after a two-week absence, though, of course her return was a cause for some sadness as it meant that more treatment was required. We joked about my having to contain my excitement upon seeing her. It is amazing, the relationships that can sprout up so quickly and vanish just like that.

The third week I drew with Andrew we made a collage for the "friendly nurse" — butterflies coming right off the page. We both signed it. Later, as he worked on a beautiful free drawing of an island and the palm trees and the sun he said, "My mom will be going home on Wednesday." "That's great," I said. His face didn't change, "I won't see you again." I stayed on his mom, "So she's feeling better?" He smiled and said, "Yeah, she feels great. I won't see you again." I thought about saying, "I will be here if you need to come back." But I didn't. "I really enjoyed meeting you" — I hope I said. "You are so bright and courageous" — I wish I said. But I probably said nothing. "It was a pleasure working with you, Andrew," I probably said. "Take care of yourself and your mom," I must have said.

Later, as I headed for the elevator, Andrew ran up. "Michael! You're still here!" He skipped along beside me as we rounded the corner. We got to the elevator, and as the doors closed, this nine-year-old boy called out, "Michael, God bless you!"

Working with Families

AIRs frequently work with everyone in the patient's room, including friends, family and occasionally healthcare staff. A patient may be surrounded with few or many family members some of whom may be grieving, laughing, angry or frightened. They may range in age, depending on the policies of the hospital or hospice, from very young to very old. In some cultures, if a family member is hospitalized, the entire extended family will descend on the patient's room, creating a challenge for the healthcare team and an opportunity for the AIR. *The gift the AIR brings is the chance for everyone to engage in a normal creative activity.*

There seemed to be a lot of people coming in and out of Catherine's room. She introduced me to her husband and her daughter and grandson, Isaiah who was six years old. Isaiah said he loved art and would like to do all sorts of things. He began by decorating a box for his fifteen-year-old cousin who had just arrived, and then did a painting to put up in his grandmother's room. Soon his great aunt came in; she was a wonderful lady and loved the fact that we were doing art. She said it was a godsend that her niece could spend time with her mother and not worry about her boy.

Toward the end of the day, we spread big sheets of paper everywhere in the room for all the family to paint, collage or write on; it turned out to be a very colorful mural for Catherine's room. When I went in the following week, she said that when she woke at 3 a.m. and looked at the mural she felt as though her family was there in the room with her.

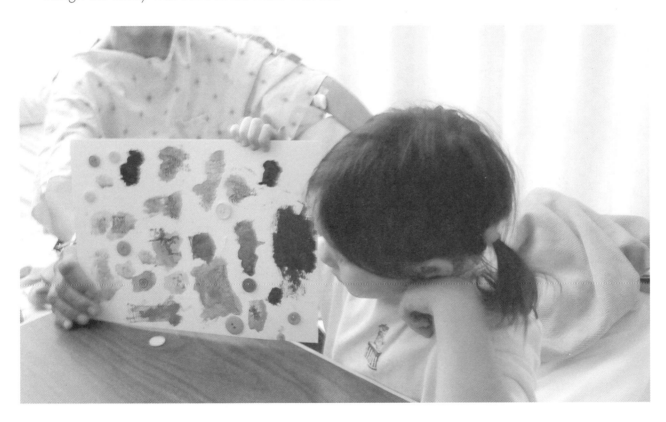

I told Theresa she could keep the colored pencils so she could have something to do while sitting with her husband. The look of surprise on her face and her pure, honest joy of receiving something so simple as a box of a dozen colored pencils was something that hit me very hard.

Victorio, who is thirty-three, has been here for a long time; he has a PhD and researches in this medical center. He has such a fresh approach to painting and drawing and is very hungry to learn and progress. It is so inspiring to work with him and so touching to see how he communicates and works with his mother. They had drawn another still life and wanted to paint it together today. It is very much a collaborative process for them. He comes up with ideas and his mother comments on them, and then they collectively draw. While one draws, the other looks on and makes suggestions. They are both becoming more comfortable with the materials — watercolor and markers are their materials of choice. I showed them how objects can be defined through light and dark rather than hard outlines, and they began to see the difference between a flat representation and a more 3-dimensional one. They work slowly and intensely together, communicating more to each other through their art than through their conversations.

Working with Children

Children are children whether they are in the hospital or at home. Because of their natural developmental abilities to become quickly absorbed in the present, they are able to move fully from having a painful procedure to making an art project. AIRs working in pediatric clinics or on in-patient floors learn to meet each child as the unique little person he or she is. This means not necessarily expecting age-appropriate physical, emotional or psychological behavior, but accepting and respecting each child's responses and feelings.

The immediacy of both the joy and the sadness of working with hospitalized children mirrors the tenor of these children's lives. Life's force is palpable as they walk through the hospital halls pulling, pushing or riding on an IV pole. Their art is often vibrantly reckless, the result of a kind of fearlessness in the face of a medium they can control. The Creative Center AIRs who work with these children consider themselves very lucky artists.

3-D projects offer more weirdness and more tactile satisfaction; kids start the project easier and censor themselves less with some of these sculptural projects. Lots of kids say, "I can't draw," when handed a large sheet of paper; but not one child has ever said, "I can't build" or make something. I like to give a theme to the project, and let the medium begin to perform happy accidents and surprises for them. Generally, kids seem to be intimidated by too many choices; I provide them with a direction that does not feel like a restraint or a constraint.

Ladies and Gentlemen, in this corner we have the reigning champion, an AIR, and in the other corner, in Room 560, we have this week's challenger, Emily! And the champ is going in strong with a friendly introduction from the child life staff. The challenger is countering right away with a firm, "No, thanks!" Oooooh! Tough blow. Will our reigning champion crumble? Wait, it looks like, yes, ladies and gentlemen, our champion is still standing and she's turning that no, thanks, into an I'll try that one. And, yes it's mother and daughter doing the art project. Daughter is complimenting mother; both are almost done! And what's this? Oooooh! Daughter crumples hers up and shoots it into the trash bin. Awwww, didn't see that coming, but mother's is coming out nicely and Yes! Daughter is hanging it on the wall! Can we make it to a next art project? The champion is suggesting it and it looks like — yes! She's got the OK! And she's back with T-shirts and fabric paint. And, it looks like, yes, ladies and gentlemen, we have a winner! Our reigning champion has turned a flat "No!" into not one, but two art projects. And the crowd goes wild —

Sicker kids end up getting preferential treatment. Is this how it should be? This is how it should be! The condition of the child is not evident in the energy or mood or the appearance of the child; it is more visible in the eyes of the parents.

Printmaking is the king of all kids' projects so far! Young kids were much more capable with this technique than I expected — also it's a good lesson in multiples. Few kids want to use mixed media! When asked if they want to add to the print by filling in blank areas with different colors of markers or crayons, no one thought it was a good idea. Not one kid wanted to add other colors; they all wanted the print to remain "pure." It is the most addictive of the projects I've done, both in the clinic and on the in-patient floor.

The Artist's Involvement — Relationships

The Creative Center's training stresses that it is the patients' interests, choices and abilities in the moment that need to be served. This is an issue that is frequently discussed in our artist support meetings when stories are told of how difficult it is to "be in the room," to stay with the needs of the patient, or on the other hand, to respect the artist/patient relationship.

A hospital is an emotionally charged environment where much of the superficiality of the "outside" world necessarily falls away. Regardless of how hard you try to respect the professional boundaries of your relationships with the patient, their families and with the rest of the healthcare staff, you will invariably find that there are those with whom you become very close. You will learn from all these relationships — some will be rewarding, others quite difficult. Many AIRs report that their work in the hospital has a definite influence on their personal work and lives. Remember that self-care is an important part of maintaining your equilibrium.

It is so hard to see Brad like this. His health has been slowly declining and it is hard to see him in this kind of pain. I knocked on his door and found him again with just a bloody t-shirt on with his head all bandaged up. There are so many sores on his body and he is hooked up to so many machines that he cannot move anymore. This scene breaks my heart and takes my breath away for the moment — I try not to show it. He said, "Hi, Rose, I'm sorry I can't do anything today." I told him not to be sorry, and asked how he was doing. When you ask this question, "How are you?" at the hospital, it is not a casual question the way we ask it most of the time; it is a real question with real answers. Since working at the hospital, I have gained new respect for this question, and when I ask it, I listen for a real answer.

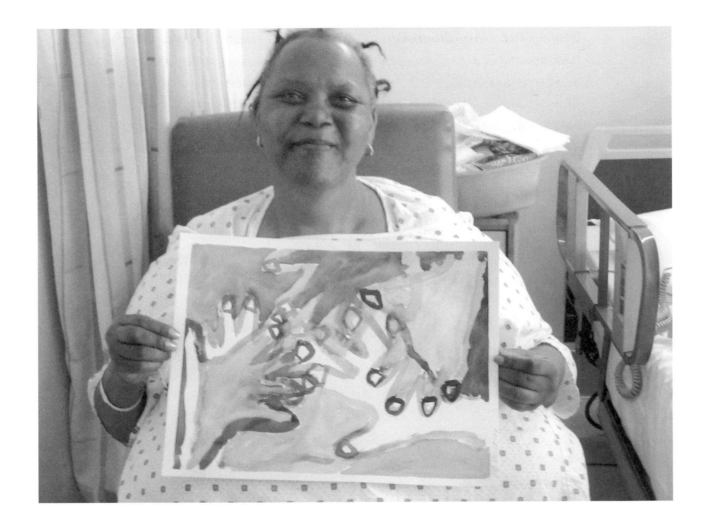

Today I worked with a woman with breast cancer. Three years ago my mother was diagnosed with breast cancer. She is alive and thus far healthy. Sitting down to work with this patient unsettled me. I could not quite shake the association between her and my mother, and my stomach was tight. We worked together for a while on a series of greeting cards, some with drawings, others collaged. She spoke very openly and comfortably about her cancer and was utterly convinced that she would overcome it. We spoke about her Bronx childhood and her grandchildren and her Thursday night card game. As is so often the case, the dread or sadness that gripped me was eventually replaced by respect and admiration. This woman was full with life, determination, a future; suddenly I saw in her the same will that I see in my mother. I didn't share any of this with her, but thanked her for it nonetheless.

Understanding Diversity

People are different from one another in a myriad of ways. An artist cannot fully engage in working with all patients and their families until she has acknowledged her own values, beliefs and ways of interacting. An understanding of how and what AIRs may contribute to those whose race, religion, ethnicity, gender, sexual orientation, socio-economic status, age, disability, language, education or nation of origin is different from their own is a vital part of an AIR's training and should be an on-going learning experience.

I showed Abdul, an Egyptian man, who told me he has five children, a book of Matisse cut-outs, including photos of Matisse working in bed and in a wheelchair. After discussing the structure of a collage composition, Abdul picked three colors and spent two hours cutting, arranging and pasting his collage with minimal assistance from me. He told me he would like to make a painting of a man with only one eye in the center of his head.

I met Damas from Santo Domingo, who has been coming for a while for treatment; she is in her sixties with a very beautiful, lined, kind face. She told me she has tumors all over her body, but that the treatment was helping her. She was reluctant at first to make a collage, but after looking at Frank Stella, she decided to try. It was the first time she ever made any art at all. She got very excited, saying this was the first time she ever did anything like this, that it was really fun and that it made her mind think differently!

She kept marveling that her mind had changed. When her infusion was over, she didn't leave because she wanted to finish the piece. Next I met Fall, a very young woman from Senegal who had been watching me work with Damas. She was very tentative about cutting and drawing, but suddenly she saw how she could make something work and was more confident in choosing yellows and violets, so I explained complementary colors to her.

Over the years The Creative Center's AIRs have learned that:

- In some cultures, life is lived according to the clock; being on time is valued over spending time with friends or family.
- Silence often indicates respect or an understanding that the speaker has been heard; in some cultures a direct "no" is rude, therefore silence may mean "no." Some cultures express an answer or thought through the telling of a story.
- In many cultures, to accept anything the first time it is offered is thought to be ill-mannered; people may expect to be asked again, and perhaps again, before accepting.
- Personal space can often be indicative of a cultural preference — standing very close or backing away may be construed as "too close or distant."
- Eye contact varies from culture to culture; it may be direct, fleeting, or entirely avoided. Contrary to European customs, avoiding one's eyes may be a sign of respect, or an appropriate behavior between men and women.
- Touch is a cultural difference that varies from the prohibition of touching certain parts of the body, such as the head or the feet, to the degree of physical intimacy that is expressed on greeting a friend or a spouse, in a public or a private place.

Those with whom we work know what makes them comfortable. If as artists, we ask our patients about their cultures, their lives and their experiences with respect and a genuine desire to understand, they will tell us how we can work together.

I had been wondering when I would see Mamum again and there she was, thinner and more yellow than I remembered her. She said that they've started her on a new and more aggressive chemotherapy, and that all her beautiful hair would fall out again. She said she needed "my art" to replace what she has lost, and began painting a watercolor of her village in Bangladesh, describing the houses, streets, fishing boats, trees and rice paddies. She said the people are so poor they eat only rice, hot peppers and mangoes; that there is no treatment for cancer there. Her painting was so colorful and lovingly done; I feel she deeply misses her home.

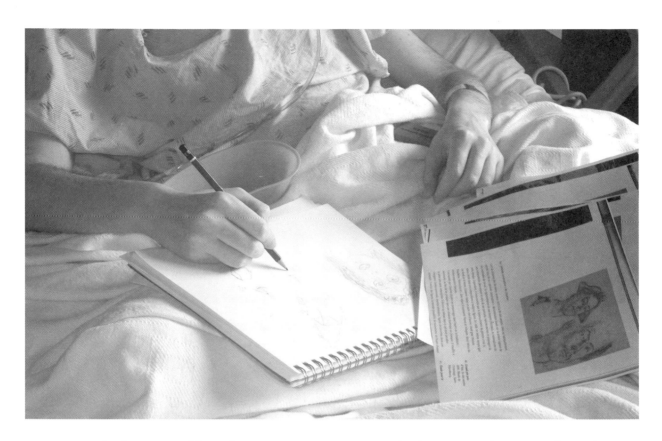

As Long as Life Exists, So Does Art

It may be that artists who choose to work in hospitals and hospices have an innately enhanced knowledge of the human spirit. Certainly, the work itself leaves no doubt that people are capable of courageous responses to the utmost suffering, and that the grace that keeps us all is found in the most desolate places.

Whether or not the artwork, or the dance or the poem, is the beginning or the end, the invitation or the response, it is the story that is often the most powerful part of the artist's and patient's time together.

What we acknowledge and believe from our work at The Creative Center, is that *as long as life exists, so does art.*

Today they told Michelle that she has extensive metastases and that they can only try to treat her pain at this point. She handled the meeting with tremendous candor and grace; she cried and asked a few questions, but did not ask how much time she has left. No one knows; she wasn't expected to live six weeks when she arrived, and she has proved them wrong. Her neck is supposedly so fragile that a sudden turn could kill her instantly and yet she has produced a room full of art and ceramics, and taught us all a great deal about perseverance and living according to one's own rules.

Waiting to go home because she did not want to die in the hospital, Betty wanted to talk about metaphysical issues; she said that after we had talked the last time, she had been trying to think of a way to express what she had been feeling lately — her sudden desires to study certain things, or do certain things, and wondering if it was bad to get excited about anything at this point. We spoke about having all these feelings and expressing them artistically, maybe in a visual journal of some sort. As she was leaving I gave her a blank accordion book that I had made. She said that it inspired her to put her feelings into some kind of format and gave her the framework she felt she needed. She thanked me and talked excitedly with the book in hand as they wheeled her out to go home.

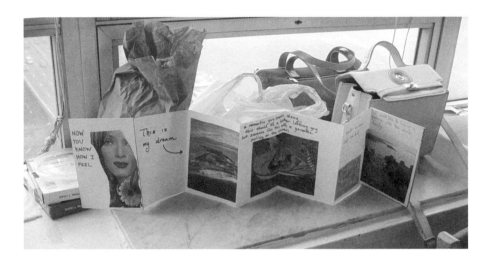

Kirsten started to open up to me a little; maybe because we were alone in her room and not working with others, but there was a level of comfort that hasn't been there before. She said, "When I was living on the street for eight years, I decorated my cart with wild colors and streamers and chimes. People loved it and I never had to beg for money; people would just like me and my cart and help me out. I have always been artistic and it always finds a way into my life." I said that I was so glad she got off the street, so she could live to share her stories and creativity with everyone here. She replied, "I am, too. I finally realized that I would die unless I got help. Bring me pictures of you, all dressed up on your wedding day. I can't wait to see them — best of luck this weekend!"

Everyone has been so excited to talk to me about my wedding. They breathe every word in deep like it is fresh mountain air. I am not sure if it is the idea of hope or if it reminds them of their own times of joy, but it seems they get a kind of renewal from it all.

She had a heavy Italian accent, wore a red bandana and was walking around the floor with an IV pole. She didn't really understand the whole drawing thing, but was willing to try. Drawing two separate flowers and coloring them in, she put down her pencil and started to tell me her whole story. The cancer — her husband's cancer, her daughter who just died of cancer, and the five children she was left with to feed and take care of. She apologized as she cried. She never complains to any one, "But what am I going to do?" She is scared, and the kids live downstairs and the grandkids live upstairs, and what is she going to do? I said, "Draw a flower for every grandchild, all five." She begins to draw; "I got more than five," she says, "I got nine." "Draw a flower for each one of them." So she draws nine flowers and colors them in; now write the names under each one.

You've got nine grandkids, three kids and a husband and they are all counting on you; maybe that's a good thing. They need you to be strong. "Can you cook?" I ask. "Can I cook? They love my food," she says, and tells me about the Sunday dinners at her house. She stops crying. "They need you to be strong," I say, and she nods her head, and has this look of defiance. Now here comes the part that always comes: "You got a wife and kids?" "No," I say. She looks really concerned. "So you live with your mother?" she asks. "No, I live alone, but I cook pretty good." She likes that, but says, "It's fine now, but you don't want to be alone when you are old and sick." "I know," I say. "You are not alone. Look at all the family you have." She starts to tear up. "I tell you all this," she says. "You don't mind?" "No," I say. "Now I see all the flowers; why not connect the flowers with stems and leaves?" She looks at me and begins to draw these abstract lines connecting the whole page. "Nice. Where did you learn to do that?" I ask. "I used to embroider in Sicily." I smile; she smiles and we hang her flower/family in her room.

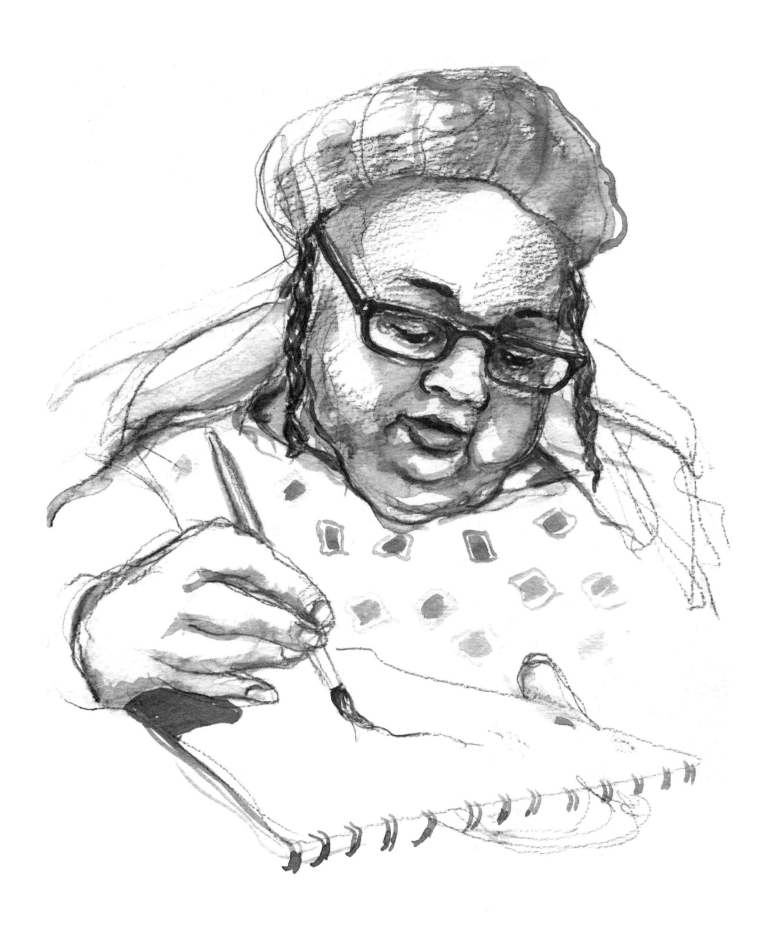

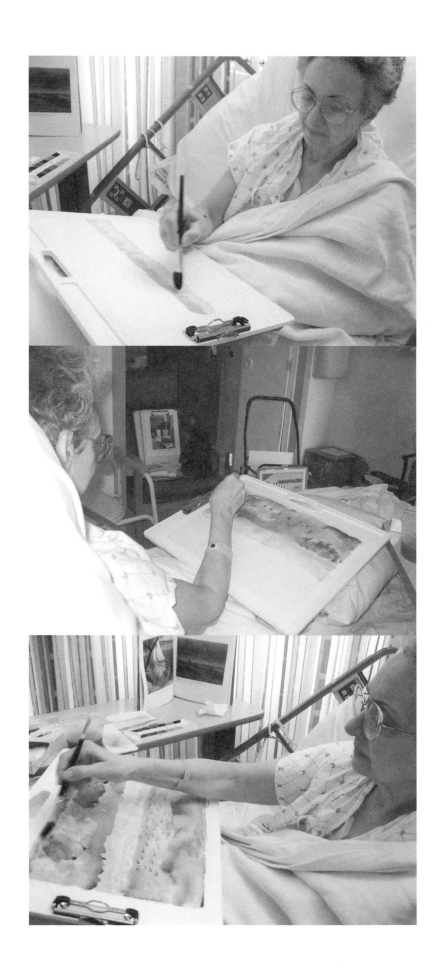

The Portable Studio

I'd stopped in Jason's room several times in the past few weeks, inviting him to paint, which he turned down each week with a different response, ranging from "No thanks!" to "Maybe next time!" Today, his retort was "I don't like to paint!" which I quickly countered with, "Well, what do you like to do?" "Puzzles!" I decided the universe works in strange ways, as I pulled out a puzzle of Monet's "Water Lilies." "Got it!"

The most important part of my job as an Artist-In-Residence is not, surprisingly, about the actual art MAKING, but "creating a space" in which to make it. I don't mean the "real space," but the space inside the patient's head and heart. The physical space can be large or small, noisy or quiet — what's important is that it is a place apart from the patient's illness and treatment. It can happen on a bed, in a chair, in the dayroom but it's the connection between us that allows us to create.

Help Wanted: an artist who can engage people to make art (who may not even know they want to) in a hospital setting (that is not set up for it) despite healthcare staff (who may not understand what the artist is doing).

"AIR," "Art Teacher," "Art Man," "Art Volunteer" — artists who work in healthcare are called many things, but their mission is the same: to bring a world of art directly to the bedsides of patients who may not even know that they want to make art! The challenge then is to find ways to present the highest quality materials, the most engaging processes and the highest level of instruction within the most restrictive of settings — the hospital. The success of the portable studio environment is dependent on one thing alone — the artist's ability to be resourceful, to "create a space" physically and emotionally, where none exists. That resourcefulness translates into flexibility — with time, materials, and creativity. Carefully laid-out materials may have to be put away at a moment's notice when "your student" is called for a medical procedure, or when lunch is rolled in early, or when a doctor comes to meet with the patient and the family. Patients may say, "No, thank you," or "I can't draw," or "I'm too sick!" — but by creating a "safe space" you will give them the opportunity to say "Yes" at another time.

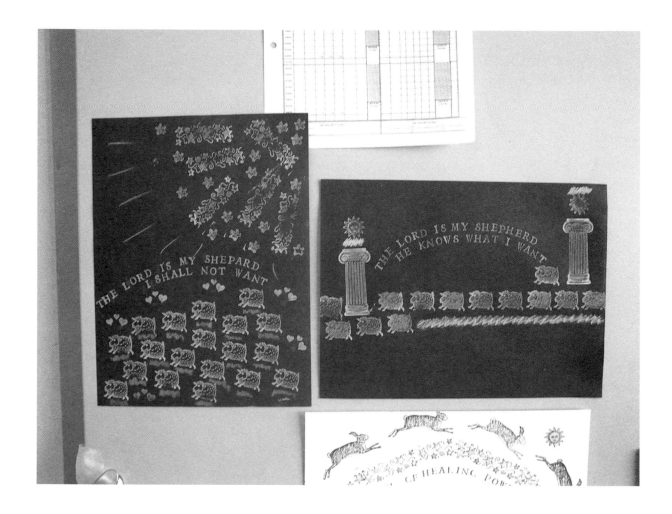

I began displaying the artwork in the rooms from the first day I started as an AIR, first rather timidly by propping the paintings on the bedside tables, and later to the wall behind the bed — but, at a patient's suggestion, I began taping their work right on the glass of the colorless prints in the room — voila! Instant framing! Everyone noticed the change immediately — the rooms became more colorful; the staff had something to chat with the patients about besides their vitals; and the patients had something beautiful to gaze at and share with their visitors. I've taught in many situations — but never in one where artmaking made so much difference!

Keeping Artmaking Simple

There are certain "basics" that apply to working with patients, regardless of the medium. One AIR begins by *making sure the patient is comfortable* so that artmaking, in no way, interferes with that comfort. This AIR works around the patient, making certain that participation will give pleasure and distraction, not become an infringement. If the patient has agreed to work in a visual arts medium, the materials should be placed in reach of the patient, next to the hand the patient will be using, for easiest access. It may be most convenient to use the patient's bedside table or the AIR may need to supply the working surface.

A stackable, ten-gallon plastic container with a flat lid (not ridged) can be used to contain all the materials you need to supply a studio in a particular medium. The lid can also be used as a working surface or lap desk. One excellent container is the "Sterilite 10 Gallon Tote Box" (#69703-00, measuring 20.5"l x 14.1"w x 12.5"h). Stacking several containers on a luggage cart allows the artist to wheel "studios" from room to room. Individual containers can be left with a patient for a period of time. Bring **lidded containers filled with water**; the patient's room may not have a sink the AIR may use (often a patient's bathroom is off-limits to the AIR).

Other items an AIR may want to always keep on hand include a **flannel-backed plastic tablecloth** to protect bedclothes, **wipes** for clean up, a **way to display finished artwork** (simple mats, colored paper for a backing, tape) and, to keep hands clean, **latex-free gloves** (because of latex allergies, many hospitals no longer allow latex gloves).

Use the best possible materials you can afford in each medium. You know from your own artwork that the quality of the materials can affect how well they work and what the art looks like. Make a note of the brand names recommended here as price is not always an indicator of quality.

Many AIRs bring **items to set up a still life** to work from. The hospital world is often monotonous, colorless and dull, and individual patient rooms even more so — except perhaps for a vase of pale flowers, an occasional balloon and the flashing images on the color TV. AIRs are thus inspired to "bring the outside in" — toting fresh flowers and foliage, brilliantly colored fruits and vegetables, small bits of the natural world (shells, stones, seed pods, feathers) as well as "objets d'art" (crockery, cloth, global souvenirs) that can inspire both conversation and artmaking. Patients can use their bedside tables to arrange the still-life set-ups themselves, adding a personal item if they'd like. The use of a **viewfinder** (a small, pre-cut, sturdy mat) can help a patient determine the subject of a representational artwork, as well as point of view and the presentation of the picture plane.

Every Setting Is Unique

Since every hospital setting is unique, each AIR must find the best way to bring the "portable studio" to the patient. Light, space, and proximity to water all contribute to the physical architecture of the "studio environment." The artist's schedule (morning, afternoon, or evening), as well as the daily rhythm of the hospital (mealtimes, test times, visiting hours, doctors' rounds) may also affect the atmosphere and tone that surrounds artist and patient.

Storage space for art materials also impacts on the types of artmaking you can bring to the patient. Working backwards from the most "ideal" setting to the reality of the one you are working in will be most helpful in trying to accomplish your goals. Although the materials, projects and storage suggestions that are discussed here are "best," many artists find that they need far less equipment and supplies than they originally imagined. AIRs are surprised

at how a little goes a long way, particularly in an environment where aesthetics may be lacking.

Keeping Artmaking Safe

In a healthcare setting, whatever materials are used must be non-toxic; safety comes from the artist's knowledge of materials and their proper use. If you are unsure of the safety of materials you are using check with the *Art & Creative Materials Institute (ACMI)*, an international association with over two hundred art and craft material manufacturer members. The organization's primary purpose is to evaluate and test products; those that are safe receive the ACMI certification seal. Information about individual manufacturers and their products can be found on the ACMI website *(www.acminet.org)* or by mail:

Art & Creative Materials Institute
P. O. Box 479
Hanson, MA 02341-0479

Some hospitals are sticklers for safety and require the artist to document the non-toxicity of the materials by providing Material Safety Data Sheets (MSDS), available from the product's manufacturer. If you are ordering from a catalog, ask if they have the MSDS for the products you are ordering. School supply catalogs are great sources for non-toxic materials.

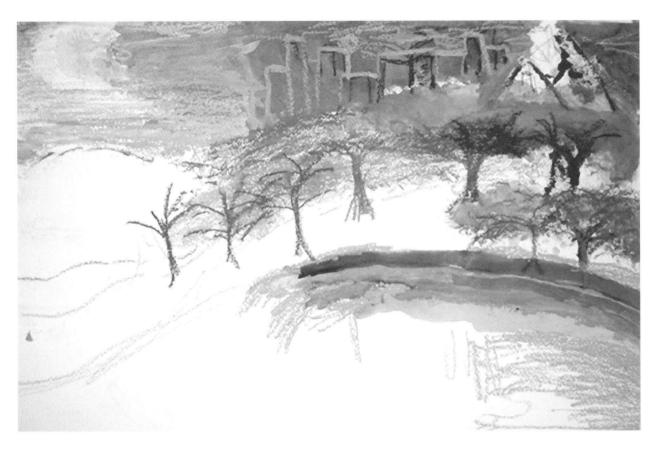

Common sense says to AVOID using the following:

1. Anything marked toxic.

2. Art materials containing potentially toxic materials that can be easily inhaled, ingested or absorbed through the skin, i.e., chalk pastels, charcoal, certain glues and some clays.

3. Solvents. Use water exclusively.

4. Razor blades, X-acto knives, scissors with sharp points and any other sharp objects.

5. Latex gloves cannot be used in many healthcare institutions; patients and employees may have latex allergies.

Ending the Session

Artmaking sessions sometimes end prematurely: a medical test must be performed; a doctor enters to discuss treatment; a visitor arrives. More often, however, a patient's stamina will determine the length of the session. AIRs need to be sensitive to the (sometimes) subtle signals that will indicate the end of your time with a particular patient. A slow-down in conversation, complaints about pain or tiredness, and visible signs of sleepiness need to be noted. Conversely, there are patients who would happily continue for a number of hours making it difficult for you to leave. Some AIRs prepare gallon-size Ziploc bags containing inexpensive watercolors, a brush, a small baby-food jar (very stable with low water capacity in case of spills) and a variety of papers clipped to a small board to leave with patients who are reluctant to say goodbye. This "gift of art" can be a significant one to patients who must face the rest of the day alone. A promise to check back in with a patient before you leave for the day will often motivate patients to continue working.

Before you leave, find ways to display the work — even damp paintings can be taped directly to the wall or mounted on small cardboard folding screens to be displayed on the bedside tables. Black construction paper makes an instant "frame" for small flat art. Ready-cut mats and double-stick tape create a professional presentation. Many hospitals establish a "patient gallery" in the hallway, the nurses' station or the family room. Clear Contact paper can be applied to the front and back of dry paintings, drawings or prints, creating a usable placemat for the tray table. One AIR provides pre-stamped manila envelopes so patients can send artwork to family and friends — right from the hospital. Many take digital pictures of the patient and his artwork. (Appendix E contains a sample

release form that must be signed by the patient if you plan to distribute these photos.) These images can be compiled to create a portfolio for AIR use (always helpful when program refunding is at hand) or can be printed and used by the patient in a variety of ways (note cards and stationery). Nurses are delighted to have a keepsake of a favorite patient, especially if it's inscribed to them, a reminder that their patients are more than their diseases.

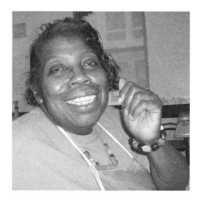

The remainder of this chapter discusses *painting and drawing,* visual media used commonly and successfully by AIRs, and *art appreciation,* a way to involve the reluctant. Examples of other media (printmaking, collage and mixed media, modeling clays, book arts, fiber arts and jewelry) are discussed in detail in Appendix G. Use all of these suggestions as a starting point. Keeping the safety of the patient foremost, *your work in the hospital is limited only by your, and the patient's, imagination and creativity.*

Painting
Why paint in the hospital?

The freedom of the painting process is the perfect antidote to the restrictive hospital environment. *The very essence of painting is choice.* Beginning with the materials one chooses, the brush one holds, the colors used, the marks made, the design and composition of the line and form — painting is ultimately a reflection of the desires of the painter. Helping patients realize those desires is the goal of the Artist-In-Residence and, with that in mind, the portable hospital painting studio should be crafted to allow patients to both identify and execute those goals.

What you need

1. A *Masonite clipboard or a piece of matboard with binder clips:* to hold paper, or that paper can be clipped or taped to, and can be left with a patient.
2. A *variety of brushes:* synthetic and sable, flat and round, hake (wide) and sponge brushes. Bamboo brushes for Chinese brush painting (be authentic!).
3. *Painting tools:* small sponges, combs (cardboard and plastic), corks (for stamping), small scissors (for making shaped paintings), small disposable plastic plates and plastic palette knives for color mixing, paper towels, wet wipes, dampened sponges placed in Ziploc bags, eye droppers for ink blots.
4. *Paper:* Buy the largest size you can comfortably work with in the hospital.

An assortment of cold and hot pressed paper is helpful in demonstrating different watercolor techniques. In addition, pre-cut Strathmore heavyweight paper, in postcard or greeting card size, may entice reluctant patients to paint a thank-you card for staff. Heavyweight rice paper for Chinese watercolor and brush painting can create a mood of serenity and beauty. Asian-inspired paintings may be glued to thin dowels (or chopsticks) and hung with red cord (for good luck) transforming the hospital room into a gallery.

5. *Paints:* In pan watercolors, we like the quality of Yarka and Prang, though Crayola has the best cerulean blue. If using semi-moist paint, let the pans dry without lids at the end of the day, making sure you wipe them clean first. Liquid tempera works well if pre-poured into muffin pans that have a plastic air-tight lid. Pour only enough for one patient. Fresh paint (stored in small squeeze bottles) can be poured on top of used paint. Tempera cakes offer the opaqueness of tempera with the ease of pan watercolors. Use them in muffin pans, pouring a little water into each pan — use the "soup" for transparency and the block for heavier, denser work. Sumi ink (or black tempera block in a plastic storage container) is for Chinese brush painting. Dr. Marten's inks have brilliant, transparent color.

Getting started

Painting, unlike some other art media, requires at least a little set up before the painting session can begin. While the AIR is doing this, patients can be thumbing through reference materials (art books or journals, art postcards, nature magazines) that can be focused on the particular art "lesson" the AIR wants to teach. Bear in mind, of course, that the patient may have an entirely different lesson in his/her

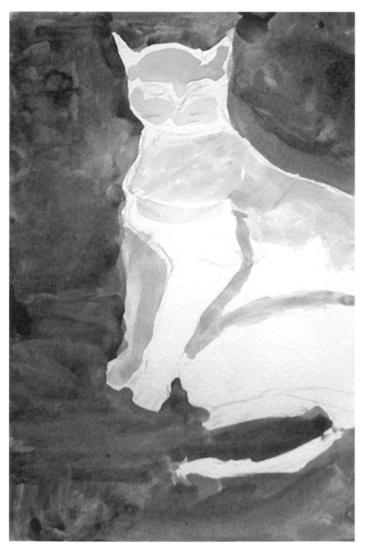

mind! These art references can be used as inspiration, or can act merely as icebreakers or conversation starters.

Many AIRs start by doing a mini-demo lesson, demonstrating two or three techniques, including brushstroke and line. One AIR uses the opportunity to teach tonal studies on pre-gridded paper, while others work in a more informal style, painting with the patient on the same sheet of paper, or working simultaneously, in call-and-response fashion, "I've made a wide line — what will you do?" or "I'll begin with red — how about you?" Still others think of the painting as the accompaniment to quiet conversation, much like music, with one affecting the other. A patient who misses her cat, for example, might like to paint a picture of her cat, or an abstract mood piece about the cat.

Once a patient has agreed to paint, the AIR has several decisions to make in guiding the painting. Will this be a skills-based painting session or a mood session? Will you offer advice on "going deeper," or will you follow the lead of the patient? Will you suggest content, such as "visualize a place you'd like to go to" or "how about painting your favorite foods?" If there are visitors, are they offered a set up as well, or does everyone work on the same paper? Does the AIR work on his/her own painting while the patient is working? *There are no rules, only spontaneous decisions that are influenced by the situation.*

When I entered Mr. Katz's room, it was dark and he was curled up in a fetal position. It was clear that his condition had worsened since the last time I worked with him. I approached his bed, and he opened his eyes. "Hi, Mr. Katz, I brought the Bonnard book I told you about." I took it off my cart, opened it to a random page and held it practically in front of his nose. "How about that blue? Did you ever see such a vibrant color?"

I took out the watercolors, and right in front of his face painted a wide swath of blue across the paper. He immediately became more alert, and tried to prop himself up with his incredibly thin arms. The nurse's aide put a pillow behind his head, and slowly, without words, Mr. Katz "painted" by pointing weakly at the paintbox and indicating where I should make the mark on the board. I finally got him to take the brush by purposely "misunderstanding" his directions. He died two days later.

Drawing
Why draw in the hospital?

Drawing is one of the most intimate art forms — using the most minimal materials, an artist can create a work that is highly realistic, fantastical or abstract. Drawing trains both the hand and the eye. In fact, some artists view the drawing tool as an extension of vision, i.e., what the eye follows, the hand traces. Drawing requires concentration and it is this concentration that allows the patient to forget his/her surroundings. Drawing is also the medium that many patients absolutely refuse at first — "I can't draw! Ask my brother, he's the artist!" — recalling their humiliation in the school art room as children. Yet many patients readily accept a pencil — it is a familiar object. Typically, adults who haven't drawn since childhood begin at the spot where they left off — for women, it is usually a house with a chimney, a waft of smoke, an apple tree and perhaps a rainbow. Men depict ships (sailboats or tankers), aircraft (particularly bombers) and occasionally dinosaurs — the world of ten-year-old boys. Under the guidance of an AIR, these images of childhood quickly give way to more elaborate drawing projects that combine developing artistic ability with subjects of importance to the patient.

Drawing is easy to set up, requiring few materials. This leaves lots of time for conversation and patients can be

I thought I would try something new and taught a drawing class to Leslie similar to those I participated in when I first learned how to draw. Our session was one of the most successful I've ever had with a patient — we didn't get bogged down in a difficult conversation, which in the past has left me feeling ineffective and sad. Leslie seemed truly engaged with what she learned and I felt confident and excited about the skills I was teaching. From now on, when I enter a patient's room, I'd like to introduce myself as an art teacher and particularly a teacher of observational drawing. Of course, I'll be flexible whenever necessary — if a patient has a particular interest or wants to work with a certain type of material I'll be happy to change my program.

left with drawing tools to continue on their own.

What you need

1. *A Masonite clipboard or a piece of matboard with binder clips:* AIRs with limited space find that artist's clipboards work well with a sketchpad clipped to it. Masonite clipboards or matboard with binder clips to clip or tape paper to may be left with patients.

2. *Individual drawing kits* can be assembled in Ziploc bags with a Pink Pearl or kneaded eraser, a small pencil sharpener, pencils in three degrees of hardness, a .5 Micron pen (for line drawings) and a fine point brush marker (to imitate reed pens).

3. *A variety of drawing materials:* Crayola Magic Markers (not the washable kind that will smear onto hands and bed coverings); Sakura Cray-Pas oil pastels (box of at least 16);

colored pencils; Prismacolor watercolor pencils; Crayola crayons (box of at least 64); and Acquarelle watercolor crayons.

4. *Paper:* Heavyweight drawing paper (90 lb. or more), at least 9" x 12" that will accept all media, is a good basic place to begin. Heavyweight Bristol board can be cut and folded to turn drawings into 3-D landscapes or constructions. Shaped manila paper may be cut into fan shapes, crowns, visors, bracelet lengths or accordion folded. Other interesting drawing surfaces include pre-cut "playing cards"; adhesive 3" x 4" labels for bookplates; heavyweight vellum; and accordion folded booklets (see section in Appendix G on book arts). Many AIRs carry small sketchpads to leave with patients.

5. *Other drawing tools* the AIR might wish to stock are small scissors to cut or shape drawings; scratching tools (orange sticks, toothpicks) for "scratch-art"; ultra-fine permanent Sharpie markers (for drawing with watercolor washes); metallic gel pens (for use on black paper — very special!); glitter pens; fluorescent markers; calligraphic pens; glue sticks; and tape.

Getting started

Many AIRs approach drawing as a "teachable" skill and will offer "lessons" in a particular area — gesture, contour, tone, composition or line — as a way to begin. The immediacy of the stroke (and the ability to change it by adding to it or erasing) can have patients feeling very successful, very quickly. Although most adults will say, "I can't draw!" they are almost always amazed at how quickly they progress when given good instruction, lots of time and quality materials. Pain and fatigue are replaced by absorption and determination as the drawing itself becomes positive reinforcement for intense concentration.

Emphasizing playfulness over skill, *drawing games* are useful to involve reluctant patients. A favorite café game of the Surrealists begins when a paper is folded into thirds and the patient draws a head of any type in the center of the top third. That is folded back and the next artist (perhaps the AIR) adds the body then folds that portion out of view. The final third is passed to another person, or back to the patient, to add legs then unfold and reveal. This is a perfect drawing activity when there are visitors to include.

Small flip books can be created by the patient: each page has a simple drawing of an animal created in any drawing medium. When the book is filled, the pages are cut in half or thirds horizontally, giving the reader the ability to "mix and match" — a perfect gift for a child or grandchild!

Full-page *close-ups of people* from magazines can be cut in half. Glue one piece on a drawing paper and ask the patient to complete the drawing. Or *photocopy works by well-known artists* (Van Gogh and Matisse are favorites) and ask patients to copy them — upside down! They will be amazed at the results. *Pre-cut decks of playing cards* stored in small bags are perfect for patients who'd like to design their own set of "heroes," "famous people" or "favorite foods."

Drawing naturally lends itself to a myriad of *mixed media projects* as well — a perfect way to "sneak" drawing skills in! Card making (note cards, pop-ups, postcards) can combine collage and drawing, perfect for those who feel they "can't draw."

Writing text in an artistic way is a great icebreaker with reluctant patients. Working with felt-tip calligraphy pens, patients can be encouraged to "embellish" the text to the point where it becomes a drawing. Using the metallic pens, letters of the alphabet can become miniature illuminated manuscripts to use as cards or bookplates. Favorite recipes can be written on index cards with decorated borders depicting food or the event, tied with a ribbon. Before they know it, patients are drawing!

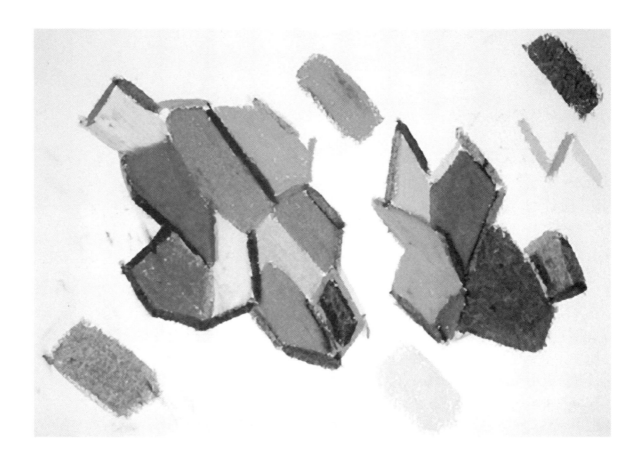

Betty was totally in awe when I showed her how to use the viewfinder to frame out the vase of flowers on her windowsill. She spent a lot of time moving it back and forth to get long views and close-ups. She looked at the flowers dead center, and in a corner of the frame — and then switched the mat from a vertical to a horizontal view. It was as if I had changed the world for her — shifting her focus in this little space made it seem much richer, much grander.

Art Appreciation —
Talking about Works of Art
Why talk about works of art in the hospital?

AIRs report that while some patients may not want to *make* art, almost all of them can become engaged in a conversation about a reproduction of a painting or photograph in the form of a print or postcard. Some AIRs prefer to carry coffee-table-sized art books which can be thumbed through or left for the patient after the AIR leaves.

Looking at art offers the hospitalized patient an opportunity to "look and look again" — for time is not an issue. By using a series of open-ended questions, *the inquiry method,* the AIR can lead the patient deeper into the artwork and encourage a longer conversation. The world that is created through these discussions will often start with the image, blossoming as the patient finds points of connection from his or her own life.

Begin by asking, "What do you see here?" This simple question allows the viewer to list all the things he or she sees. "What do you think is happening?" is the next question which gives the patient the chance to begin telling the very personal story that he or she sees. The artist can interject, "Why do you say that?"

asking for evidence from the art itself, *the looking again,* or from the patient's personal experience.

Although narrative realist painting and drawing, and documentary and street photography are easy for patients to relate to as they tell the story, abstract art can work equally well. Focusing more on form, color, line and composition, the same questions can be posed. The "What do you see here?" often elicits comments about how the work makes one feel, and "What do you think is happening?" lends an anthropomorphic twist — "I think this little orange line wants to be very close to the blue one, but the green one won't let him!"

Talking about artwork is a very new and exciting experience for most people — all comments are allowed; all experiences are viable. This is a true *anything goes!* experience, particularly when juxtaposed with the neutral hospital setting.

What you need
1. *Good quality reproductions:* interesting prints, postcards, images from magazines and calendars (mounted on board). An artist portfolio with clear plastic sleeves is perfect for holding an array of artwork for discussion.

2. *Art books* with color reproductions or high quality black and white photography work well, as do catalogs from art auction houses.

3. *Museum postcards*: many museums will give you the slightly damaged cards they can't sell — you, in turn, can leave them as gifts for the patient.

Getting started

Many AIRs use art prints or books as conversation starters while they are setting up the bedside studios. However, using the inquiry approach with very little "art historical" information given about the work and based on open-ended questions designed to look harder and go deeper, discussions can comprise the entire visit. These discussions are driven by the patients, not by what experts have decided people should know about specific works of art: "How do you think the artist felt when she painted this?" versus "Don't you think the artist felt sad?"

There are three types of questions one can use to talk about works of art:

1. *Factual questions* have only one correct answer as in "What color is the boat on the left?"

2. *Interpretive questions* can have more than one answer, but the answer should be supported by evidence that's presented in the artwork — "I think that this painting shows the early morning because of the way the light is reflected on the window." People can respond differently to interpretive questions — "What is the woman on the grass thinking?" It's important to ask interpretive questions that build on one another so patients have to refer back to the artwork.

3. *Evaluative questions* ask for beliefs, opinions or points of view — there are no wrong answers. The answers can combine prior knowledge, experience and mood or intuition. This form of questioning is a great way to connect with hospitalized patients, allowing them to relate the art to their own lives.

A good website to learn more about inquiry-based questioning is *www.youthlearn.org*. The tenets of the model are easily adaptable to working in the hospital with either children or adults.

Creating Your Portable Studio

These suggestions, and those in Appendix G, are places for the AIR to begin. You will develop your own style of working with patients and create your own portable studios of artmaking materials. The important thing to remember is that your work is about the patients — what will interest and distract them, what will be safe and, if you're lucky, what you can teach each other about art.

In the past month I have worked with Arthur, an African-American prisoner who is receiving in-patient chemotherapy treatments for cancer. He is about thirty-five years old and grew up in Harlem. When I first met him, he was excited to have contact with someone who is not medical personnel nor from the prison system. Other than some drawing in grade school, Arthur had never made any art, nor was he familiar with any art terminology or history. In our first session, I asked him if he would like to look at some art books with me and talk about art. He had already told me that he couldn't do any art himself; he was too self-conscious about it. I chose the Bill Traylor book and used an inquiry method to engage him in interpreting the images and to understanding about Traylor's life. He was fascinated with the historical aspect of the work, the photos of the artist and the fact that Traylor was an untrained artist who had been a slave. Although the police guards outside his door were suspicious of me and kept coming in to see what we were doing, we spent two hours talking about Traylor's artistry, vision and use of symbolism. When I left he begged me to come back the next time he would be in the hospital, which I assured him I would do.

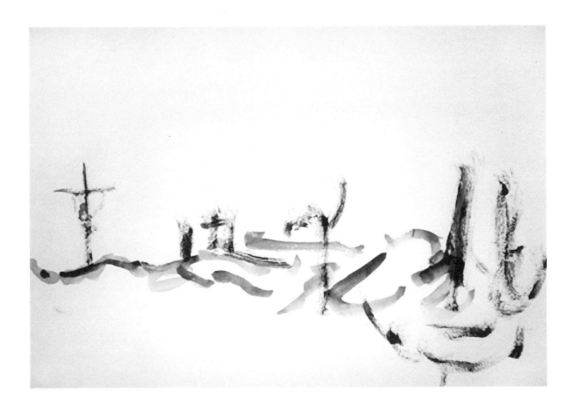

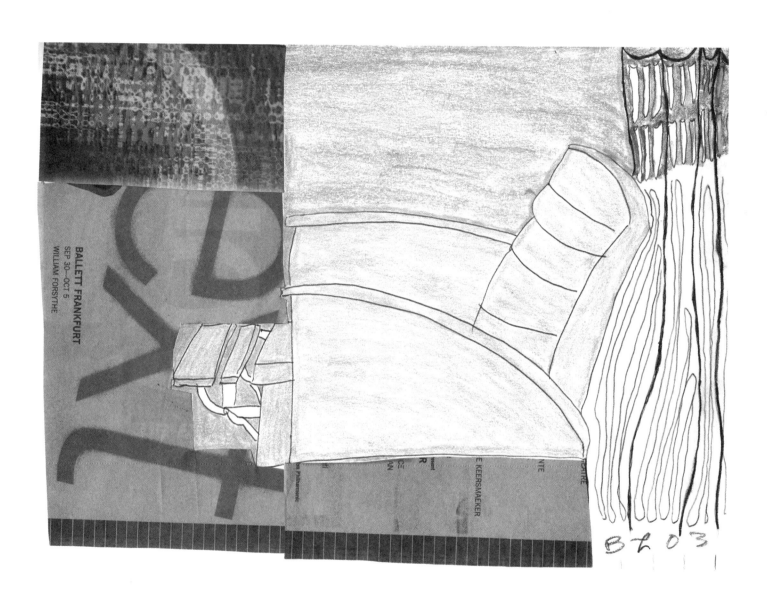

Caregivers and Caregiving

Natasha's sister calls while I am working with her and, in a fiery, funny dialect Natasha tells her to stay away from a man who has been desperately courting her. When she hangs up the phone, Natasha delivers to me a loud, hysterical harangue about men and their courting ways, about all the mistakes she's made in her life, and about her little sister and how she loves her and wishes she would smarten up a bit. She has me doubled over laughing. I leave, feeling pale and timid and dried up in the face of Natasha's passion. She may have more soul than I. How have I lived as long as I have and known so few people like her?

When I went in to see Terry today I was amazed at the number of small sculptures he'd created during the week. He showed me each one and then told me a long story about how his wife had come to love classical music because her bird enjoyed it. He then said, "You've permanently impacted my life. I don't like TV and there's nothing else to do here. Now I have all of this." He also showed me drawings of a castle he hoped to make once he'd finished the menagerie of animals for his wife.

Rewards of Caregiving

A *caregiver* is anyone who provides assistance and care to someone in need, often over a long period of time — not only medical, nursing and physical help, but also companionship. The caregiving experience can be as rewarding for the caregiver as for the cared-for.

Caregivers may be divided into *formal*, paid professionals and paraprofessionals, and *informal*, unpaid family and friends. Professional caregivers include physicians, nurses, therapists, Artists-In-Residence and social workers. However, the vast majority of paid caregivers are paraprofessionals —

nursing assistants, home health aides, nurses aides and personal care assistants. Informal caregivers, family and friends, provide 70–80% of the long-term caregiving in the United States.

Caregivers' Stresses

Many professional and paraprofessional caregivers say that they initially chose the field of healthcare because of a strong internal calling to serve. Unfortunately, physicians and nurses who trained in the past were encouraged to value intellect, rationality and stoicism above empathy, subjectivity and vulnerability. This "disconnect" may take its toll by desensitizing and isolating healthcare staff from their emotions.

Informal caregivers are caring for someone they love who now needs their help. This role may have come to them without preparation or warning. Established relationships often shift and change. There may seem to be no end to giving in this challenging situation and these caregivers can start to feel the effects.

Caregiver Burden and Burnout

It has been well documented that caregiving, both by formal and informal caregivers, has the potential to be very stressful when the needs of

caregivers go unmet as they strive to serve the cared-for. Common among caregivers is the sense of "losing one's self" — the potential danger of giving in to self-neglect, exhaustion, apathy, anger and even depression. *Caregiver burden* is the name given to the multi-faceted response to physical, social, psychological, emotional and financial stressors associated with the caregiving experience. When caregiver burden progresses to the point that it is no longer healthy for caregiver or cared-for, the caregiver has reached a state of *burnout.* The caregiver may have neglected his own health and personal needs, and lost his sense of identity outside the caregiver role.

Signs of burnout to watch for in professional and paraprofessional caregivers include job dissatisfaction, substance abuse, cynicism and withdrawal from or over-involvement with specific patients and families. These caregivers may experience chronic fatigue, insomnia, bodily aches and pains, lower energy levels, less enthusiasm and a failure to manage basic life-maintaining activities.

In informal caregivers, signs of burnout may be seen as increased sadness or depression, altered sleep patterns, change in appetite, excessive worry and anxiety, and increased use of prescription medications. Their most frequently reported unmet needs are finding time for self, keeping the cared-for safe at home, managing emotional and physical stress, and balancing work and family responsibilities.

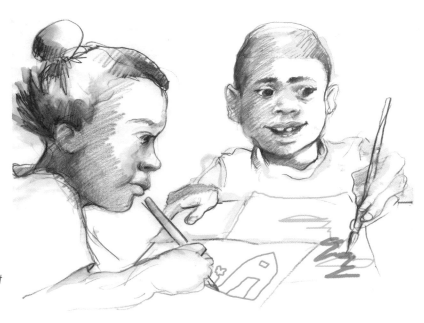

I've been here almost a year now. I think I am starting to get a bit burnt out. I may be avoiding bedsides again. The playroom is lighthearted, but the bedsides feel heavy lately. Maybe it's me. The patients who need bedsides are the ones who are in the most pain and danger...well, the children in the playroom can be in just as much imminent danger...death and suffering lurking in their futures, but they are happy at the moment. Art and the fellowship of hanging out with other children is enough to bring them joy for the moment.

The bedside patients are suffering now. I can't not think about it and I've begun to notice that I actually do spend a lot of mental energy not seeing the scars and the tubes and the needles and the shunts and the bandages. I don't really know what to do with the information when I do see it, so I try not to. I'm useless...

I know art is useful because it gives children a realm of autonomy free from the constant "Do this, do that" that they get from parents and doctors. It provides an escape from whatever physical and mental issues they are dealing with. Plus creativity is just plain fun...but I don't feel useful. I feel useless. At least at bedsides. There's so much pain and suffering and it's not fair and I can't fix it, and I can't not see it right now and the more I notice it the sadder I feel, because I really really really do wish I could do something about it. I was a lot better at being emotionally detached when I first started, but I guess it's catching up with me. Hmmm maybe I would feel better if I cried from time to time...stopped holding the sadness in and just let it run through me. I suppose it wouldn't hurt anybody if I cry from time to time after I get off work...yup, I do feel better.

Caregiving for the Dying

Caring for someone who is dying can be an incredible opportunity and experience, though also difficult, stressful and sad. People at the end of life often focus on relationships, creativity and spirituality, and frequently are able to let go of the mundane details that occupy others. A receptive, empathetic caregiver, attuned to a dying person, is privileged to bear witness to the journey that each of us will eventually, inevitably, take.

Nikhil, the lovely and elegant man from India, held his hands toward me. I had hoped and truly thought he was not going to have to return, but he is obviously very sick now and can hardly speak. He wrote his wishes and questions down on a paper that he had at his side. He had made cards before and wanted to make two more, one for a daughter's birthday and one for his son's graduation. He could not attend the birthday or the graduation and was heartsick about both. Many of his children work in this hospital and one who works in surgery came by to attend to him. She was impressed to see the cards he had made because she knew he didn't have the strength. I told her I made them but under his strict instructions as to what he wanted and where to place the stickers. I also had to write a lot of nice things on them from their dad. Nikhil always greets me and says goodbye in the Indian tradition of his hands as in prayer and with a nod of his head. His daughter thanked me for doing this kind of work and expressed gratitude for what we do. I wonder if these cards would be the last gifts they would ever receive from him and if this is the last time I will see his long, slender finders in the form of a prayer, which is the Indian way to acknowledge the humanity in us all.

Caring for Caregivers: What Can an AIR Do?

Patients are not the only ones in healthcare needing "creative attention." The premise behind *caring for caregivers* is that individuals must first care for themselves, in a holistic manner, before giving to others. Both the caregiver and the cared-for need to lead full lives of their own.

Fundamental to caring for a caregiver is supporting that individual's self-care efforts. Artists-In-Residence can offer creative self-expression and the arts as opportunities for self-care and self-discovery. Just as AIRs work with patients to help them engage their creative processes, in a similar manner, artists can offer creative outlets to both formal and informal caregivers, rejuvenating body, mind, emotions and spirit — rebuilding resources depleted by caring for another.

AIRs work at the bedside with families, as well as with patients, offering the same collage, drawing, painting, poetry or writing activities to everyone in the room. Or, the AIR might set up an open studio in the waiting room and help family members make something to hang on their loved one's hospital room wall. In some institutions, cancer patients and their families have painted ceramic tiles that then become part of a healing wall. Other healthcare facilities hold painting workshops on acoustic ceiling tiles, installing the hand-painted tiles in the hospital's ceilings in public areas. *An AIR can create a normal experience for family and friends, allowing caregivers and the cared-for to spend time together productively and meaningfully — to make non-illness-related memories, to enrich communication and stay connected to their creative selves.*

In addition, AIRs may hold workshops or create projects for groups of formal caregivers. Even a short watercolor break during the night shift can allow nurses to relish a few rejuvenating minutes. Holding an arts workshop for staff is a good way to get to know the patient care team and to gain their trust and support for the work you do with patients and families.

Alison, the social worker, was celebrating her birthday, so I had made her a card during the day, and Luz and her family (one of the patients I had worked with) actually made her one as well. A busy day that ended with so much love and generosity.

Coming down the hall I was stopped by a young woman who asked what I do. After I explained, she asked me to visit her mother in a nearby room. When I introduced myself, the mother didn't seem interested. Her daughter persisted, however, and asked for some watercolors. Since the mother didn't want to paint, the daughter painted some flowers for her. We talked about coming to this hospital and how overwhelmed they both felt. The daughter said she wanted to continue to paint for a while and would drop the watercolors off later. I said, of course.

Caring for caregiver programs can be more extensive. At one hospital, an artist partnered with the nursing retention specialist to have the nurses write a book about the nursing experience, helping them remember what originally called them to nursing. The book was published and given to the nursing staff (from RN to aide) during Nurses' Week. "Days of Renewal" at a large university medical center integrates the creative arts with other holistic health modalities in a day-long program (offered many times yearly) to teach techniques of self-care to formal caregivers (nurses, social workers, therapists, mental health counselors). Some institutions sponsor annual employee art exhibitions and theatrical reviews or facilitate on-going writing or reading discussion groups. For the AIR who approaches situations with a creative bent and looks to the arts for a means to involvement, surveying the healthcare institution may spark caring for caregiver ideas.

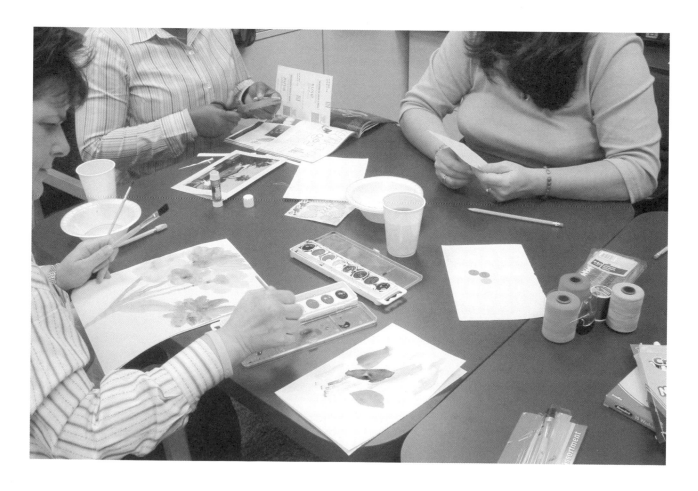

Today was a special day…a break from the routine. I had prepared a workshop for the nurses and I was nervous about how it would be received. Over the past two months I have learned that they are extremely busy and under a great deal of pressure. Barbara, the nurse manager, and I went back and forth, in person and via email, exchanging ideas for the workshop. It was decided that I would help them make jewelry boxes. Each person was provided with a small craft box and paints, glitter, markers, paper and other "notions" to use for decoration.

I brought what I thought was going to be an excess of supplies — but it really ended up being just the right amount of boxes. Barbara had arranged lunch, so we negotiated the spaces for both the art and food in the small room. I was curious to see how these overworked nurses would be able to take a break and make art. Several were just too busy — they said a quick hello, grabbed some food and ran out again. Others were able to find someone to cover for them while they sat down and created a box. I spent my entire day there which gave me the chance to be available for all the lunch breaks for the daytime staff. I worked with nurses, nurses aides, nursing students and other staff. It provided a wonderful forum for interaction — not just between them and me — but for them with each other. Some people really took their time decorating their boxes; some kept coming back whenever they had a chance to work on theirs. I was impressed not only with the talent, but also with the diverse ways that people chose to decorate their projects. I was surprised to hear how many questions they had for me about the work that I do with patients.

The day was over all too quickly. Before I headed out, I had gathered quite a bit of feedback. I walked away knowing that I would be much less anonymous the next time I walked through the halls of 16E.

How AIRs Care for Themselves

Establishing reasonable boundaries for your hospital work will help you maintain your equilibrium and be a more effective caregiver.

1. You are there to *meet the needs of the patient* — to offer choices, and make art.

2. When you feel overwhelmed, leave the scene. *Do what helps you regain a balance.*

3. *Observe all hospital rules and regulations;* remember you are there to work as an artist not as a medical employee.

4. *Give the patient's visitors priority,* even if you are in the middle of making art.

5. *Respect the patient's confidentiality.* Only repeat something said to you if you feel the patient is a danger to himself. Then tell him that you are reporting to the staff. Any other discussions with staff about what you and the patient have discussed is gossip.

6. You may become close to certain patients over time. It is generally prudent to *withhold personal contact information.* If the patient feels she must have a way to reach you, give her your supervisor's number.

As you help patients and caregivers find creative outlets to meet their self-care needs, *remember to care for yourself.* Good artists are highly sensitive and empathetic. You may find yourself experiencing the feelings similar to those described in caregiver burden and burnout. Talk with other AIRs; check to be sure you are observing your boundaries; write in your log. Work with yourself; use your particular creativities to recenter and rejuvenate.

Caregiving Takes the Efforts of Many

To care for a patient takes the efforts of many caregivers — individuals who also have needs that must be met to ensure the best possible environment of care. Caregiving for people with illness is stressful. One can find many lists of suggested self-care methods (doing things one enjoys, pampering oneself, eating healthy food, laughing, talking to others, getting time away, journaling and finding strength in faith). *The AIR makes a valuable contribution by providing activities which not only involve caregivers in their own creative processes, teaching them a skill which can be returned to, but which often results in artworks — reminders of time spent creatively in self-expression.*

I'm still learning how to do this. I come in and out of self-consciousness as I sit with patients. Sometimes the sessions are all auto-pilot, uncalculated flow, and unfettered sincerity. Other times I am working to methodically achieve results step-by-step: ingratiate myself, establish a rapport, coerce the patient into working with me, maintain their interest, enhance their mood, conclude with lightness and optimism. In a purely clinical way, I am just one more in the battery of treatments deployed by the hospital against the ravages of Cancer. In every other way, I am a person trying hard to help another person.

Working with the Dying

I knew Elizabeth was in the advanced stages of cancer. But for a minute it was hard for me to grasp that the woman I had seen engaged in making a painting on April 16th, my birthday, had died two days later. A few long moments had passed and I heard the director say, "It was good you worked with her," implying I had brought something good to this recent stranger who had taken hold of part of my heart. Continuing, she said compassionately, "That's why I tell you that when you're working with someone it should be as if it's the last time you will be seeing them."

Dying and death are normal processes that are part of the life cycle, and certainly part of the healthcare experience for some patients and the AIRs who work with them. Whether the AIR works in a regular hospital setting or in a facility that is specially designed to help the dying patient be more comfortable, work with people at the end of life is different from working with others.

Juxtaposed with a sense of urgency to bring art to someone who may not live much longer, AIRs who work in hospices often talk of the pleasure of working with the same patients over a course of weeks or months. Hospices accept patients who are in the final six months of life (although they may live longer). An AIR has the opportunity to work in a more elaborate and focused way — helping patients (and often family members) to create an artwork slowly, or to learn skills and build a large body of work, something not possible when working with briefly hospitalized or clinic patients.

When I arrived today Lester had already started a painting and there was another of his in the lounge. Then I found a collage that he forgot about. Luckily, I had my scrap pile with me and I got to work helping him finish it. I'll take it home to varnish and mat, and I'll bring it back for him next week.

Susan is such a radiant person, still so full of life…it bubbles right out of her…we always have such stimulating conversations…so I steered it towards artists today and she just took off running on O'Keeffe, Khalo, Duchamp, Klee and Kandinsky. I started painting as we discussed them. I showed her what I was doing and gave her a paper and brush, tilting the palette so she could see the colors…It wasn't a big effort, but it **was** *a painting, an introduction to the endless possibilities. I can't wait until next week!*

Learning about Dying and Death

An AIR who works with dying patients requires knowledge, wisdom and sensitivity to end-of-life cultural beliefs, physical changes and emotional needs.

Cultural beliefs

Each patient is culturally unique. Whatever culture we are part of has influenced our attitudes, beliefs and fears about dying and death. It is important for the AIR to keep a willing ear, open mind and accepting attitude in acknowledging what, in an individual's cultural background, is significant in this context.

Maureen broke into tears shortly after I arrived asking if I thought cancer was a punishment from God. She said she'd always tried to be a good woman and just didn't understand how this could be the end of her life. I did my best to simply support her and let her talk about her disappointments, losses and feelings. She briefly hinted at her anger and then apologized profusely for crying and "not doing this right." All I could tell her was that there was really no right way and she was welcome to cry or do whatever she wanted to. She then said she wanted to "get on with it" and work on her mural project — "it's too empty and I've cried enough today."

It was a quiet visit but I also was very aware that there just aren't enough gentle ears and perhaps I had offered enough to Delores just listening to her say "I'm dying" and acknowledging what she had to say.

The physical process of dying

Understanding what will occur during the dying process is basic to everyone involved in patient care. The goal is to make death better — to make the experience of dying as comfortable as possible for patient, family and healthcare providers. Addressing all the needs of the dying person is essential. Through the arts, an AIR can offer a type communication and self-expression that, while unfamiliar to many people, can remain meaningful to family, friends and providers long after the patient has died.

Terminally ill patients, who do not die suddenly, begin a process that involves specific physical changes. These changes generally start one to three months before death occurs. The actual dying process often begins within the two weeks prior to death. In many, a shift occurs that takes them from mentally processing death to a comprehension and understanding of their mortality.

Often I'm surprised by how long some people live while their bodies are terribly deteriorated. Cancer is an unpredictable creature wrapped in hope, loss, grief, revelation, anger and acceptance. It does feel epidemic here. It's a potent reminder to live my days fully.

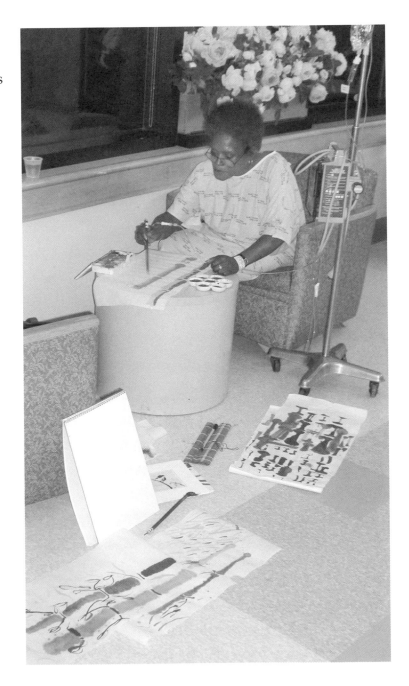

June 2: I received a referral to work with John. When I walked into his room I immediately noticed that this man, who was so incredibly thin, was sitting straight up in bed having an animated conversation with his brother and father. He told me about his love of art and we had a rollicking conversation about art and art history. At one point we were talking about depictions of death in art. Quite frankly his family looked shocked but John seemed relieved and vibrant.

July 8: I went upstairs to visit John. I hadn't seen him last week since he had been with medical staff both times I went to his room. He was noticeably weaker, his skin sallow, his elbow as bloated as a cantaloupe in contrast to his cachetic body. His eyes were open, and moving slowly, erratically, but he did not seem to notice my knock or entrance into his room. I have learned to go close to people at this stage and to talk gently and clearly to gain their attention. "John? It's Melanie." He smiled and then lolled back; his eyes again wandered, half closed. He "came to" again and talked clearly for a moment saying how nice it was to see me before saying, "It's hard, my mind just comes and goes." His brother and father arrived. I went over to John and suggested that I should go. "So soon?" he asked; I told him I didn't want to interrupt his family visit. He slowly pulled his hand into the air and I gave him mine. "Thank you." he said, kissing his fingers and gesturing toward me. I didn't say I'd see him next week. I'm not sure that I will, but we both said thank you and goodbye.

July 22: John died last week. Actually many if not most of the people I have been working with have died in the past few weeks. It's become a different experience to check the weekly census and see who has "expired." I now hold my breath, hoping for some that they got their wishes to let go and be out of pain and for others that they got theirs to stay alive.

The scenario will vary greatly according to the cause of death, the person's general health, medications and any other significant factors. The AIR can expect to see some or all of the following changes in a dying patient:

One to three months prior to death:

- *Withdraws, loses interest —* first from the world (newspapers, television), then from people (friends visiting) and, finally, from loved ones.
- *Sleeping increases —* more naps and time spent with eyes closed.
- *Words lose importance;* touch and wordlessness take on more meaning.
- *Loses interest in nourishment —* nothing tastes good; liquids preferred to solids.

- *Weakness increases* — overall energy declines.
- *Experiences hallucinations, illusions, delusions* — consciousness fluctuates, vision and hearing changes.

One to two weeks prior to death (the physical body is losing its ability to maintain itself):

- *Sleeps most of the time,* but still responsive.
- *Picks at bedclothes* and has agitated arm movements.
- Is *disoriented and confused.*
- *Body temperature lowers* by a degree or more and can fluctuate between fever and cold.
- *Skin color changes* becoming flushed with fever and bluish from cold.
- *Pulse rate is erratic.*
- *Blood pressure begins to fall,* gradually.
- *Perspiration increases,* often with "clamminess."
- *Circulation to the extremities* is diminished so that the hands and feet begin to feel cool compared to the rest of the body. The nail beds on hands and feet become pale and bluish rather than the normal pink.
- *Breathing changes* from a normal rate and rhythm into a new pattern of several rapid exchanges of air followed by a period of no respiration.
- *Congestion can occur,* a rattling sound in the lungs and upper throat as air moves across accumulated phlegm.

Just days to hours prior to death:

- Sometimes the person has a *surge of energy.* They may talk clearly, ask for food, visit with relatives.

The one to two weeks' signs become more intense as death approaches:

- *Restlessness increases* due to lack of oxygen in the blood, or there may be no activity.
- *Breathing patterns are slower* and more irregular; may stop for 10–15 or even 30–45 seconds before resuming.
- *Congestion* can be very loud.
- Eyes may be open or semi-open, teary, but with a *glassy, un-seeing look.*
- Hands and feet are purplish. The knees, ankles, elbows, and undersides of arms, legs, back and buttocks are blotchy. Skin color may change to pale yellow pallor or a dusky, darker grayish hue.
- Finally a *coma ensues* and may last from hours to minutes before death occurs. Persons in a coma may still hear what is said even when they no longer seem to respond to verbal or even painful stimuli.

Death has occurred when the person's heart is no longer beating and there are no signs of breathing.

The emotional work of dying

Loss causes us pain. *Grief* is the personal experience of loss. Everyone grieves in his own unique way. The patient grieves the loss of health; the family, the loss of a loved one; both, the future they had anticipated that is not to be. Through the pain and hard work of grieving, we come to terms with what has changed our life and how our life has changed. As best we can, we accept, cope and learn to live with our loss. All grief is not alike. A significant loss may change one person forever; another person may rebound quickly. There is no right or wrong way to grieve; no schedule to follow.

Psychiatrist Elisabeth Kübler-Ross was one of the first to describe the five *stages of grief.* Anyone experiencing any kind of loss may move back and forth, with varying degrees of intensity, among some or all of these stages. Each step aids the healing process. It is helpful for the AIR to be aware of the changeable emotions that may be encountered while working with patients and their families.

- *Denial* — "This isn't happening!" Denial is a protective emotion when a life event is too overwhelming to deal with all at once.
- *Anger* — "Why is this happening?" Physical activity may help one deal with bursts of anger.
- *Bargaining* — "If I promise to do, say or be 'x', then 'y' will happen." Guilt is a primary emotion in this stage.
- *Depression or sadness* — "I don't care anymore." At this stage the loss can no longer be denied and that realization causes a profound sense of sadness.
- *Acceptance* — "Things are just the way they are and I can't change them. I'm ready." Some resolution to the loss has taken place; adjustments have been made and it has been incorporated as part of life.

Grief and hope can coexist. There is much a dying person can hope for and experience. Dying patients may resolve issues that they had been unable to previously and/or find greater understanding in the meaning of life. Caregivers often share in hopeful experiences while witnessing another's dying process.

Emma and I decided to test combining her crayon drawing with watercolors. As we worked, she decided she liked the crayon alone better — at least she was open to experimenting. She is so ill, but she told me that she believes life can always be open to change and new beginnings.

Today I met with a seventy-four-year-old man who was just told he had only a short time to live. He had a wife, two children and three grandchildren. For nearly two hours we talked about his life: how he met his wife; what he had learned from his son; why he should never have retired from teaching. He thanked me for letting him talk about his family. It was all he could do to elude total despair. I waited an hour or so before seeing another patient. I'm still thinking about Daniel and what that conversation meant to me, and him.

Mr. Kim was eating today when I went to visit but was happy to get the instructions for the origami model he'd requested. He talked about dying for the first time and trying to get things in order for his wife as he folded and unfolded the paper. Before finishing he said he was tired but asked me to come next week to work on the flying crane model again.

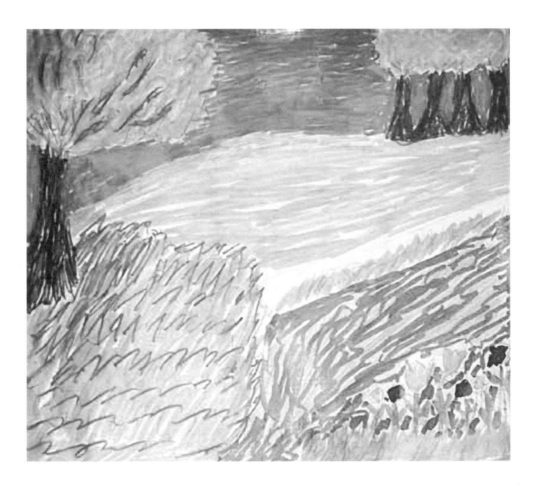

Working with Children and the End of Life

The children an AIR will work with could be family members of someone terminally ill, or the child himself may be dying. Each child will have her own unique perception of death, influenced by her age and level of maturity, and by the beliefs and fears of the family. It is important for the AIR to understand that children mature at different rates and those who are ill or highly stressed often regress to earlier levels.

Children of all ages (and adults as well) need honest, consistent and accurate information. However, if the subject of death arises while you are working with a child remember that your job as an AIR is to help him make art and that your best response is to be a good listener. If you have concerns, talk with the social worker or nurse manager.

Children communicate their concerns and fears in many ways; the AIR can offer a range of age-appropriate art materials and projects to encourage self-expression. Being sensitive to each situation, AIRs should do what they do best — provide opportunities for children in difficult situations to create.

I worked with Adam, who was too sick to come to the playroom today. He is very, very ill but he really wanted to work with me. When I bent the wire, he made a sword — and he kept going. Then he made another — two swords: one for him and one for whoever was going to fight him.

Something scary did happen this week. Sam started bleeding and got quite a lot of blood on his shirt. Fortunately, he was okay with it, really calm. It had something to do with his abdominal IV. It seemed like this had happened to him before. They changed his shirt, but I felt like a real dork because I had walked up to him and asked if he wanted to work with me — he'd been looking right at me. That's when his father showed me that he'd bled all over. I feel like this job has some complex emotions going on. I waver between the silly, productive, joy of art and the mortality of these kids.

A Time for Palliative and Hospice Care

Palliative (supportive) care is care in which the primary goal is one of comfort rather than treatment and cure. Here, medical treatment emphasizes pain relief and symptom control for patients. The goal of palliative care is that no person should suffer through an illness or die alone or in pain. Palliative Care is a new medical specialty that provides the prevention of and relief from suffering, including the suffering associated with a terminal illness.

When a person with a terminal illness ceases to respond to curative treatments, he may choose *hospice care*, a type of palliative care in which the patient agrees to forgo curative and life-sustaining treatments (though he may change his treatment plan at any time). Hospice care emphasizes the control of pain and discomfort while still treating the symptoms of the disease. The focus for the patient and family becomes the emotional aspects of care; medical concerns no longer dominate.

The goal of hospice care is to keep the dying patient as alert and comfortable as possible in a familiar environment by relieving physical symptoms, giving physical assistance and supporting the patient's and family's emotional, social and spiritual needs. Hospice means "place of shelter"; care occurs in the patient's home, nursing home, hospital or hospice center. Hospice teams are comprised of physicians, nurses, social workers, dietary counselors, physical therapists, pharmacists, aides, chaplains, therapists, trained volunteers and AIRs.

An AIR has much to offer as part of a hospice care team — helping the patient and family create artwork that will, undoubtedly, hold special meaning. The AIR may work with the patient and all family members. For the dying person, what he creates with the AIR could be one of the last things he makes; it often becomes a very important remembrance for the family. For family members, making something for the patient helps them overcome their feelings of helplessness and brings a sense of normalcy into a difficult situation.

The Arts, a Gift at the End of Life

The gift that the arts and an AIR offer to a dying patient is an expressive way to live until the very end of life — to enjoy time, to create, to leave a mark — to be engaged in the now.

*Dean was awake this week when I went by to see him. "I'm a dead man,"
he said. It was even more difficult to understand his speech and he didn't
have the energy to work hard at communicating so we did our best for a few
moments. He asked about the weather outside saying he really didn't notice it
anymore and then told me about Christmas. It was a short visit and I know that
we probably won't have many more. But before I left he said, "Just come" and
indeed I will.*

*Betty was also notably sicker and did not wake when I went to visit. I did
spend a few minutes with her husband though who told me she was very proud
of her autumn tree mural. He wants to make sure that he is able to take it home
when the time comes.*

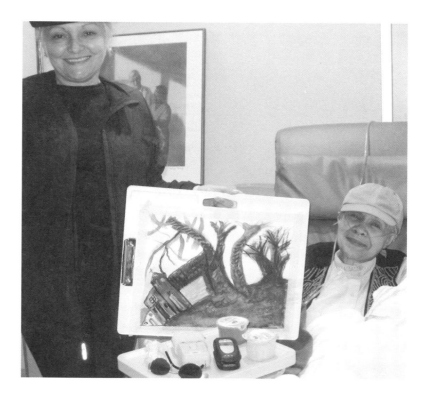

*Sometimes I worry about the art that isn't being made in the time I spend
with Lucia and others, yet this is just the ebb and flow of this hospice and of
living with cancer. I've placed the desires of the individual above my own
interests in making art, glad that perhaps I'm the one person in the hospital who
can and will follow the patient's agenda. Just as I have learned and flourished
as an artist and a person through this experience, I see the patients I co-create
with as wonderfully unique people — alive and growing in their own ways.*

Getting the Word Out: Communication!

The nurses, social workers and doctors were visiting and asking the artist/ patients about what they were doing, how it worked and admiring their artwork. It's great when art can change the hospital dynamic a bit and encourage practitioners to interact with people as individuals rather than as patients, illnesses and cases.

It's not enough to do great work — people, both inside and outside the healthcare institution, need to know about the Artist-In-Residence program. Building knowledge of and support for the program will help the arts be a valued and expected part of the healthcare experience. Just as the artist works to cultivate support from the patient care team, so should she communicate with the institution's public relations department. Ideally they will help you contact those within the hospital and also in the community interested in learning about your efforts. Public relations knows that publicizing your good work will also make the institution look better.

Basic Marketing and Advertising 101

A hospital is a competitive business. As such, it markets itself for the same reasons a grocery or discount store does — to foster relationships with its customers and the community; to build brand recognition; to differentiate itself from its competitors; to increase top-of-mind awareness; to attract new customers; and to enhance the loyalty of existing customers. Because healthcare institutions are often large and employ hundreds, if not thousands, they are also concerned with building relationships and maintaining the loyalty of their employees, volunteers and referring physicians as well.

There are two kinds of advertising: paid and unpaid. *Paid advertising* includes the ads consumers encounter on TV and radio, in the newspaper, on bus benches and billboards. It is also when hospitals pay to sponsor events such as golf tournaments, charity benefits, symphony performances, etc. Paid advertising keeps the hospital's name and programs in the public eye in ways the institution can control. *Unpaid advertising* includes news stories in any media and word-of-mouth. Unpaid advertising has a greater perceived value, so employees in the community relations department work hard to maintain a good relationship with those in the media. Interesting stories are beneficial to both groups. If the artist provides a good experience to patients and their families, they will tell others and more people will come to that hospital — that's good word-of-mouth advertising.

Working with Marketing and Community Relations

Whatever the hospital's department is called, Communications, Media Relations, Public Relations, Community Relations or Marketing, these are the employees responsible for promoting the "face" and "feel" of the institution. An AIR needs to work through a hospital's established channels. Introduce yourself to this department. Let them know what an AIR does; let them know you are willing to provide publicity. If you have a brochure about your program, leave copies with them. Get the name of the person you should contact when you have an interesting story. Each

hospital has its own policy on media contact; be sure to find out what it is at your institution. Any photo of a patient or staff member must be accompanied by a signed release form before being used. Your hospital can provide you with copies of theirs. And, there is our sample in Appendix E. Remember to always respect and protect patient privacy.

Many hospitals pride themselves on having a "healing environment." The work an AIR does is human interest about patients and/or caregivers. Often a particular patient or a special project is a newsworthy story — one that could be shared — one that defines the healthcare experience in a unique way.

Getting the Word Out
Inside the institution

Most hospitals have systems for publicizing internally the interesting things that are happening within the institution. Find out what these ways are and use them to let those in the hospital (patients, staff and visitors) know about your program. Submitting an article to an internal newsletter is a good way to introduce yourself, offer tips for creative activities for caregivers, talk about a successful program, etc. Many hospitals have bulletin boards that change periodically; an AIR might offer to design one about the program. Look around your institution to see what ways those who are there connect with one another. *Remember: the more who know about your program, the better!*

Outside in your community

Supporters for your program can be developed in the community as well. An AIR can consider establishing an advisory board made up of persons interested in the arts, healthcare and fund-raising. Speaking to civic groups and having a booth at community events educates about the value of arts in healthcare (as well as the caring, progressive, enlightened nature of your hospital). Local high schools and universities may be good sources to provide possible interns and

volunteers. Other healthcare- and arts-related agencies, as well as your state's arts council, may be interested in becoming involved in an Artist-In-Residence program. Individuals you meet and educate can help the program grow in many ways, from assistance with fund-raising to providing a base for volunteers.

Create a Network of Support

A passionate, knowledgeable AIR is the best person to take responsibility for creating a network of support within the hospital and throughout the community. Continual communication is one very good way to help an AIR program flourish and grow.

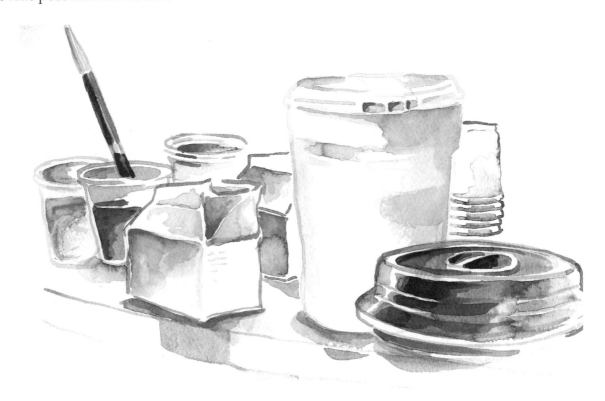

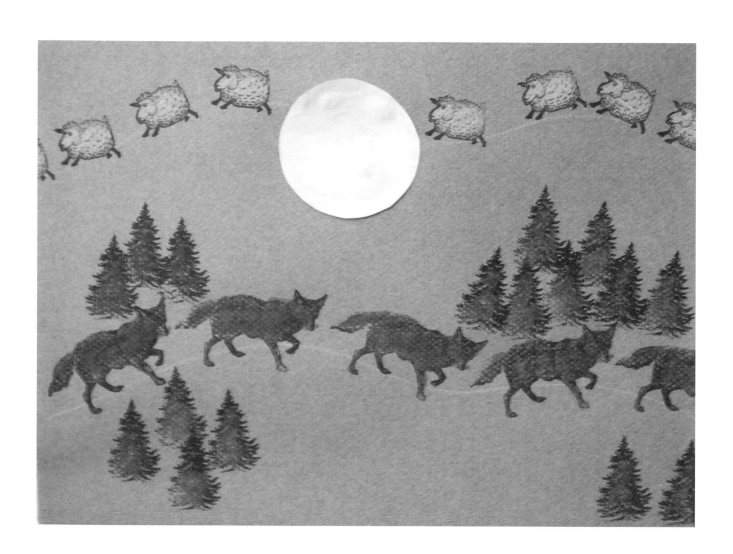

Evaluating The Creative Center's Artist-In-Residence (AIR) Program

When the physician prescribes a medication, one of the primary ways in which he or she evaluates whether or not the medication has worked is to ask the patient. *Self-report* is a direct, cost-effective way of finding out what works. In the field of arts in healthcare, this direct approach is sometimes overlooked as research analysts adopt the rigorous medical model of quantitative evaluation.

Because the mission of The Creative Center is to bring the individual experience of artmaking as a gift to patients to lessen their anxiety, pain and fear, we discussed whether or not filling out evaluations and answering questionnaires would interfere with a patient's individual choice to work with an AIR. As the number of funding organizations that required program evaluations as part of their granting process increased, we applied for a grant that would enable us to conduct a non-intrusive study of the benefits of our Hospital AIR Program.

Formal Evaluations: Grant-funded Studies

The Creative Center received an initial grant from the United Hospital Fund to develop and implement a year-long evaluation of our AIR Training Program. In 2002, The Creative Center received a follow-up grant. This second grant, The Satisfaction and Outcome Assessment Project, identified the results of artmaking with an AIR (outcome variables) and developed and implemented measurements of patient and staff (consumer) satisfaction with the AIR program in five of the eight hospitals where our artists then worked. In gathering data from patients and hospital staff, the interviewer focused on the patient's experience of making art and on the staff's perception of the patient before and after artmaking

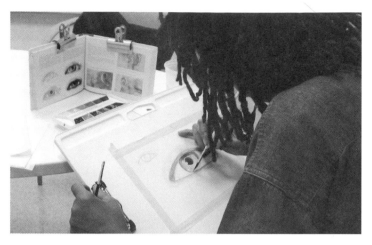

with the AIR took place. *Over 92% of the patients, when asked their overall opinion about the AIR program, said that it was a "good" or "great" idea.* 84% of staff replied that the program appeared to make patients more optimistic or cheerful. The assessment established a baseline measurement of the satisfaction so that further data could be collected and compared on an on-going basis.

This study facilitated the artists' clearer understanding of patients' expectations and needs, and enhanced the artists' ability to enrich the environment of the hospital staff. Taken together, the two studies continue to facilitate The Center's evaluation of our AIR Program.

Informal Evaluations: Logs, Visits, Meetings

The work of our AIRs is constantly being evaluated informally through The Center's supervisory process of written logs, individual supervision, site visits and AIR group meetings. The AIRs write logs that chronicle each of the days that they work in their hospitals (changing all patient and staff names to ensure confidentiality). The logs help the AIRs to integrate their work as they reflect on their experiences, and keep The Center's staff up-to-date with the work each AIR is doing. Staff also make periodic site visits to observe the AIR at work.

Every six weeks all the AIRs gather over supper at The Center with the staff. These group meetings enable the artists to discuss their challenges and questions with one another — an important part of what can otherwise be an isolating work experience. Practical art ideas are exchanged, patients' memories are honored, and both personal and professional thoughts are shared.

Using the Results

The on-going results of both The Creative Center's formal and informal evaluations have helped the AIR Program remain responsive to patients' and healthcare staff needs and requests; enabled the AIR Program to flourish and expand based on its strengths as well as the demonstrated need; and provided the artists with increased knowledge and a great deal of pride in their work.

Having a Creative Center AIR in Your Community

After having read this book, studied the photographs and learned about our Artist-In-Residence Program, we hope that you share our vision that *art is a creative experience — making art, talking about art, looking at art — and should be an enlarging, nourishing, enriching, healing part of everyone's healthcare experience.* And we hope you share our belief that *medicine may cure the body, but art heals the spirit.*

The goal of The Creative Center is to enable *more artists* to make *more art* with *more people* in *more hospitals and hospices.* We have shown that in working with our AIRs, many people were making art for the first time and they took enormous pride in what they had made — creative children and adults whose spirits were thriving in the face of tremendous physical challenges. Their art shows us and their caretakers tell us.

In the emerging field of Arts in Healthcare, the programs that develop nationally and internationally seem to spring from a person or persons who have a passion that they are determined to have realized. The story of The Creative Center serves as a example of how the passion, expertise and determination of two women has grown and developed into an entity that has helped thousands of patients and caregivers through the arts.

How The Creative Center Began

In 1994 Adrienne S. Assail and Geraldine Herbert founded The Creative Center in New York City. Adrienne's experience as a cancer patient and singer/songwriter and Gerry's work as a social worker in a bone marrow transplant unit convinced them that art and artmaking could improve the quality of life for people with life-threatening illnesses.

At that time, support groups were available, but did not appeal to everyone; the knowledge and use of alternative medicine was still fairly covert. Gerry and Adrienne believed that women were underserved and their experience had shown them that women responded more frequently to group activities than men, particularly when faced with an illness. The two decided to find a way to offer free art workshops, taught by professional artists, to women with cancer and subsequently opened The Creative Center for Women with Cancer.

The first classes were led by artists who volunteered their time to teach skills-based (as opposed to therapy-based) classes. The workshops took place in a donated space that also served as office, art studio and gallery. The first official funding they received was used to pay the artists. The Center has never charged the participants and has always paid the artists. Their current space, an open, airy loft on West 26th Street, still serves multiple functions — studio, office, gallery, library and meeting space.

Next Developments

Many of the women who came to the workshops said they wished that artmaking had been part of their healing experience while they were hospitalized. In 1997, the first Creative Center Artist-In-Residence Program began at Lenox Hill Hospital with one

artist working with cancer patients one day a week at the bedside. Word quickly spread about the overwhelming success of this unique program and other hospitals began requesting AIRs for both children and adults on their oncology floors, chemotherapy clinics and bone marrow transplant units. In 2002, The Center began a training institute for artists and others who wished to establish AIR programs outside the New York City area.

The work of The Creative Center has continued to grow and expand — new goals emerge when a need arises and new programs are created to fulfill those goals. (Details about The Creative Center's growth and development can be found in the "Timeline," Appendix A.)

Initiating an AIR Program in a Hospital

The Creative Center's introduction to each of the AIR hospitals has been distinctly different. Typically, introductions are based on who we know, or who knows us. Rarely have we entered through direct administrative channels; more often our first contact is with someone we know who is a nurse, a social worker or trustee. Initial discussions center on the ways in which the AIR program can benefit the patients and staff of that particular hospital, and the opportunities that exist for the hospital to be able to offer an AIR to its patients.

Funding for our Hospital AIR Program is a collaboration between the hospital and The Creative Center; each is responsible for half the total cost of an AIR working one day a week for one year. Requiring hospitals to be funding partners gives them an investment in the partnership. The Center seeks additional funding partners for our share of the cost, often receiving assistance from foundations and corporate sponsors.

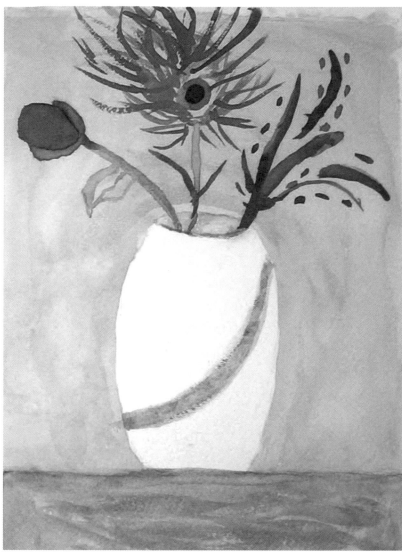

Our Successful Program

Since 1997, Creative Center Artists-In-Residence have been working in hospitals, hospices and other healthcare facilities. Yearly we serve more than 15,000 patients, their families and staff. We offer patients the opportunity to learn about and become absorbed in their own creative resources at a time that is usually filled with fear, anxiety and boredom. We provide caregivers much needed opportunities to connect with their creativity in a stress-filled environment.

We at The Creative Center have written this book and developed our Training Institute because we know that our Hospital Artist-In-Residence Program helps people and is an excellent model to emulate and replicate. Our resources and expertise are available to others who share our passionate belief *that if art is good, then it is good everywhere, and especially good in healthcare settings where the human spirit is in need.*

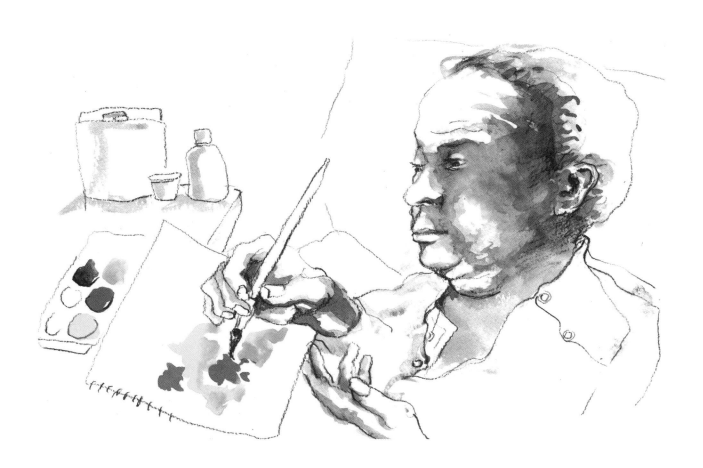

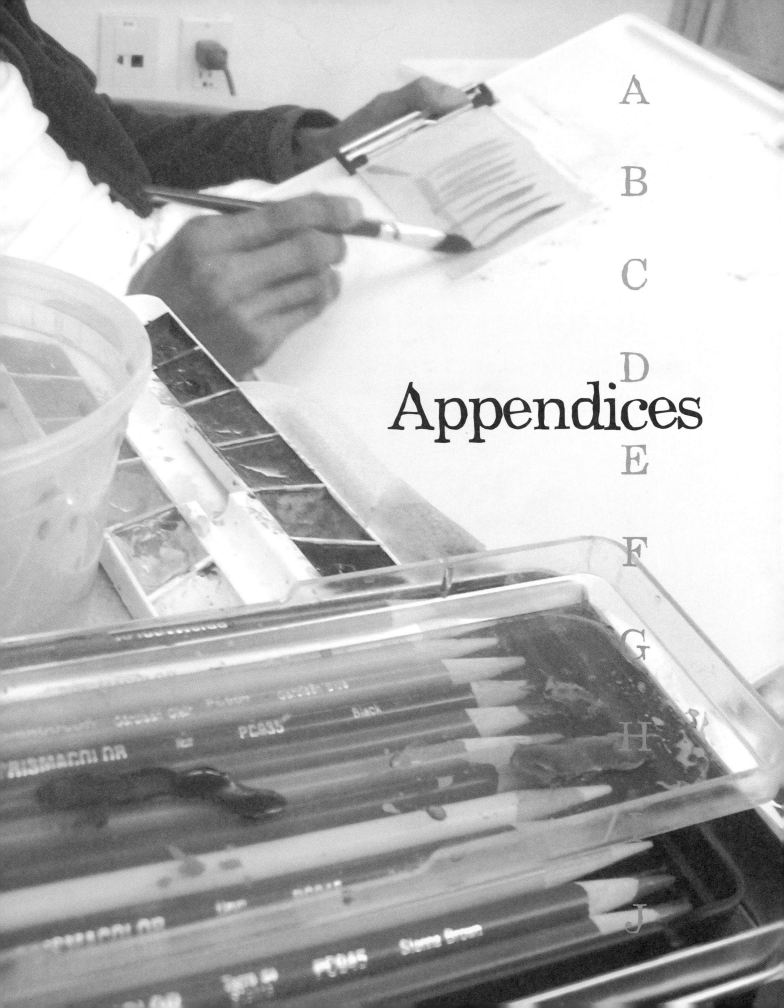

Appendices

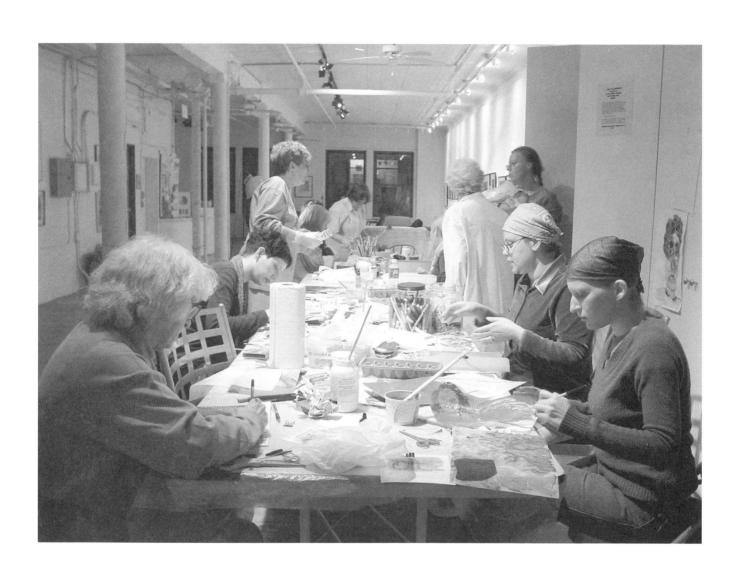

Timeline:
The Creative Center

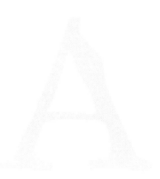

1994

Geraldine Herbert, a social worker in a bone marrow transplant unit, and Adrienne Assail, an attorney and singer/songwriter, collaborated to develop their idea of a creative "home" for cancer survivors. Initially using borrowed space, The Creative Center began as a series of free workshops in the visual, literary and performing arts, taught by professional artists, offered to women with cancer.

1996

The Center held its first public exhibits of participant and professional artwork. Venues included the ABC-TV Gallery, The National Arts Club and The World Financial Center (curated by The Whitney Museum of American Art) as well as shows at The Creative Center's in-house gallery.

1997

The Hospital Artist-In-Residence Program began at Lenox Hill Hospital — enlarging The Creative Center's mission and bringing the opportunity to make art directly to the bedsides of cancer patients.

2000

The Creative Center moved to its present location, a loft on West 26th Street, where workshops, festivals and open studios flourish; it became the home of our Gallery and a performance space for music, dance and improvisational troupes and readings from our literary groups.

2002

The inaugural Training Institute for Hospital Artists-In-Residence sponsored by Bristol-Myers Squibb, took place in May 2002. This week-long Training Institute prepares artists from around the world to work in hospital settings through seminars, workshops and hospital internships and is led by physicians, social workers, nurses, artists and art educators. To reflect the more than 5,000 men and children we had served through our Hospital AIR Program, we changed our name from "The Creative Center, Arts for Women with Cancer" to just "The Creative Center."

2004

The Creative Center celebrated our 10th Year Anniversary with our Artist-In-Residence Program operating in nineteen hospitals and serving more than 15,000 patients every year.

2005

The Creative Center continued our Training Institute, which has trained more than sixty artists from around the U.S. and Canada who continue to receive support and resources through The Creative Center Artists-In-Healthcare on-line Google chat group network and Training Institute newsletters.

In collaboration with Harvard Medical School, a course for medical students was developed called *Training the Eye: Improving the Art of Physical Diagnosis.* The ten-session course includes didactic sessions at the medical school and observation practicums at the Museum of Fine Arts, Boston.

The Creative Center hosted its second annual Colloquium for Leaders in the Field of Arts in Healthcare. The four-day fully funded conference included seminars on the challenges and opportunities in the field and produced a white paper, *Arts in Healthcare Programs and Practitioners: Sampling the Spectrum in the U.S. and Canada,* that is being distributed widely in the field.

2004

The Creative Center was awarded a two-year Lance Armstrong Foundation Community Grant for *Still Life: A Documentary Photography Project for Cancer Survivors,* a project that is enabling participants to learn the art and craft of digital photography while documenting their experiences as survivors. Participants attend classes and seminars with professional photographers and educators from The Whitney Museum of American Art and the Museum of Modern Art. Portfolios of the juried work will be published in book form to help educate healthcare practitioners, policymakers, caregivers and the general public.

Into the Future

Today, as the field of Arts in Healthcare rapidly develops, there is a great demand for educational resources and training materials. The Creative Center continues its role as a dynamic contributor. In addition to the publication of this book, *Artists-In-Residence: The Creative Center's Approach to Arts in Healthcare,* The Creative Center will continue to add to professional development in this field by promoting and facilitating the discussion and publication of materials and guidelines that contribute to the development of values, ethics and best practices.

Art in Healthcare: The Benefits are Endless

Addresses~
Psychosocial needs

Assists~
In reaching developmental goals

Builds~
Family unity
Self-esteem

Decreases~
Agitation
Confusion
Depression
Dyspnea
Loss of independence
Pain
Restlessness
Self-isolation
Social isolation

Elevates~
Emotional well-being

Enhances~
Body image
Communication skills
Decision-making
Independent living skills
Quality of life
Self-control

Expands~
Interpersonal relationships
Range of motion
Support network

Heightens~
Self-awareness

Helps~
Acquire knowledge and skills
Develop trust
Maintain productivity

Improves~
Cardiovascular functioning
Coordination
Ways of coping

Increases~
Life and leisure satisfaction
Physical conditioning
Self-reliance
Short- and long-term memory
Strength and endurance

Prevents~
Decline of health status

Promotes~
Adjustment to disability
Community integration

Reduces~
Anxiety
Stress

Sharpens~
Cognitive skills

Strengthens~
Psychological well-being

Teaches~
Vital life skills

Final Report Summary:
Satisfaction and Outcome Assessment of the Hospital AIR Program of The Creative Center 2002/2003

Patient Satisfaction

Over 92% of the respondents, when asked their overall opinion about the AIR program, said it was a "good" or "great" idea. These results far exceeded The Creative Center's stated objective that at least 85% of the patients would express satisfaction with the program.

Impact of the Program

The staff was also asked to comment on their observations as to the impact on the patients of the AIR program.

- 84% of respondents replied that the program appeared to make patients more optimistic or cheerful.
- 75% of respondents replied that the program appeared to relieve patients' boredom.
- 67% of respondents replied that the program appeared to help patients forget their pain.

Summary

- The quantitative and qualitative data indicate that patients and staff were overwhelmingly satisfied with The Creative Center's Hospital Artist-In-Residence Program.
- The data from both patients and staff also show that The Creative Center's major objectives of relieving patient feelings of boredom, anxiety, loneliness and sadness were achieved.
- There was strong evidence that the secondary but important benefit, that of making the job of the caregiver staff easier, was also achieved.
- A significant number of staff interviewed said that the patient was more willing to talk about treatment options and/or responded better to treatment after the artist's visit.
- The major suggestion for program enhancement was to expand it: more locations, more days, more hours and more activities.

Full copies of this report are available from The Creative Center.

Fact Sheet:
The Creative Center's Hospital AIR Program
Overview, Benefits and Features

Overview

The Creative Center's Artists-In-Residence work bedside and in small group settings with men, women, and children — in oncology units, bone marrow transplant units, general medical/surgical floors, intensive care/respiratory units, palliative care programs, and outpatient clinics — offering these patients the opportunity to learn about and become absorbed in their own creative resources.

Benefits

The program enables hospitals to offer their patients a multitude of benefits:

- Relief from anxiety.
- Distraction from pain.
- Respite from boredom.
- A safe outlet for their emotions.
- Extended contact with a caring and supportive individual, which can augment the hospital's patient support services.
- The opportunity to engage in creative expression, which may lead to a new appreciation of their innate ability to express themselves through the arts.

- An experience of mastery at a time when they have little control over their daily lives.
- The discovery that their own creativity may augment their coping skills by accessing resources they did not realize they had.
- Strengthened communication with the hospital staff, especially when patients' artwork is displayed and the staff has the opportunity to interact with the patient as a creative and unique individual.
- An enhanced perception of the hospital as a nurturing and healing environment.

In addition, the program has been demonstrated to increase the nursing staff's sense of pride in being able to offer their patients something very special.

Features

- *A proven program* that is working effectively in over twenty New York-area hospital sites including: Bellevue, Beth Israel, Brooklyn Hospital, Calvary, Columbia

Presbyterian, Lenox Hill, Long Island College, New York Hospital, New York University, North General, St. Luke's–Roosevelt, St. Vincent's, Terrence Cardinal Cooke Healthcare Center, Mt. Sinai Hospital and Englewood Hospital in Englewood, New Jersey.

- *An award-winning program* that has been recognized with recent grants from the United Hospital Fund, National Endowment for the Arts, Bristol-Myers Squibb, Novartis Oncology, Johnson & Johnson/The Society for the Arts in Healthcare and Blakemore Foundation.

- *A professional program* staffed by professional artists who are screened and trained to work within the hospital setting and who receive on-going supervision, education, and support.

- *A responsible program* supervised by credentialed health professionals.

- *A flexible program*, where art projects, materials and experiences are tailored to the specific needs of the hospital environment and the patient.

- *A long-term program*, in which a dedicated artist will work at the hospital one day a week for a minimum of one year as a responsible member of the hospital team.

How It Works

- An Artist-In-Residence is a collaborative venture between the participating hospital and The Creative Center. Trained Artist There is a financial commitment for the hospital which covers half of the cost of one artist to work one day a week over the course of one year and includes all art materials, professional training, supervision and consultations. To make the program financially feasible for the participating hospital, The Creative Center matches the hospital's contribution.

- A staff member at each hospital is selected as the liaison between the artist, the hospital and The Creative Center to facilitate an effective and fulfilling experience.

Contact us for more information.

The Creative Center
147 West 26th Street, 6th Floor
New York, NY 10001
Tel. 646-336-7612
Fax. 646-336-7914
www.thecreativecenter.org
info@thecreativecenter.org

Sample Release Form: Patient or Caregiver

Sample Patient or Caregiver Release Form

Out of my respect for the work of The Creative Center in bringing artists into hospitals/hospices to provide patients with the opportunity to participate in the making of art, and my desire to support the efforts of The Creative Center in making its work known to others,

I, _____ ,

(Print or type name of patient or caregiver)

hereby grant to The Creative Center a royalty-free, non-exclusive license to use photographs of me, as well as works of art or photographs of works of art created by me under the supervision or encouragement of a Creative Center Artist-In-Residence, in any Creative Center print publication or audiovisual work that serves The Creative Center in furthering its mission of bringing the power of art to patients in hospitals or hospices.

_____

(Signature of patient or caregiver)

_____

(Date)

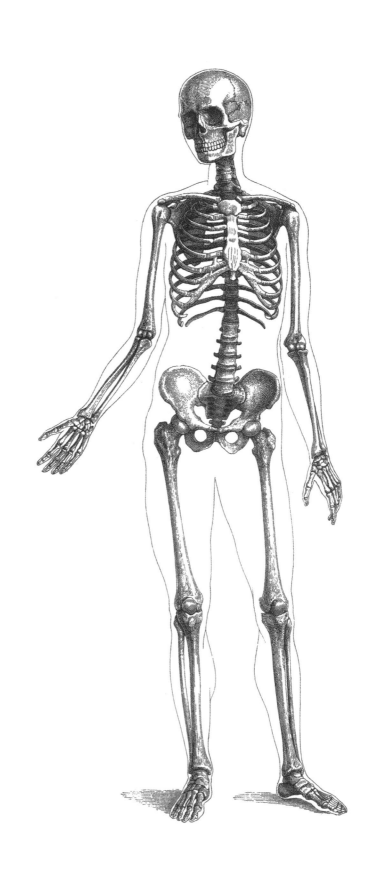

The Human Body:
Understanding Systems and Life-Threatening Illnesses

Each artist feels differently about the amount of medical and disease-related information she wants and needs to work effectively in a healthcare setting. In addition to The Creative Center's Professional and Medical Protocols, we teach AIRs about the human body and the manifestations and treatments of life-threatening illnesses. Some artists believe that additional knowledge will help them in their work and take advantage of our medical resources to learn more about a disease and its treatment. A basic understanding of the symptoms of an illness and its treatment enables artists to begin their work by immediately focusing on the individual, rather than being distracted by the medical and physical aspects of a patient's disease.

Systems of the Human Body

The workings of our bodies are reviewed in this overview of the principal systems, and the disorders associated with each. Though discussed separately and briefly, it's important to remember that *everything is interconnected and each system is highly complex.*

Skeletal system

The skeletal system is made up of the 206 bones that support and protect our bodies and anchor our skeletal muscles. The ligaments, tendons and cartilages that hold the bones together and comprise the nose, larynx, trachea, bronchial tubes and outer ear are also part of this system. Blood cells are produced in the bones' marrow.

Disorders of the skeletal system include fractures and sprains; spinal deformities such as scoliosis; degenerative joint diseases including many forms of arthritis; and bone cancer.

Muscular system

Muscles are tissues that contract. Our bodies have three different types: cardiac, smooth and skeletal. The cardiac muscle is the heart, a striated muscle, and is considered part of the cardiovascular system. Smooth muscles are involuntary and include blood vessels, intestines and lungs (all parts of other systems). The muscular system refers only to our skeletal muscles, those voluntary muscles attached to the skeletal frame that enable bodily movement by pushing and pulling the skeleton.

One common disorder of the muscular system is an abdominal hernia. There are several diseases of the nervous system (muscular dystrophy, amyotrophic lateral sclerosis [ALS], Parkinson's Disease and multiple sclerosis [MS]) which cause weakening and wasting of the skeletal muscles.

Cardiovascular system

The heart, blood, veins and arteries, our cardiovascular or circulatory system, transport oxygen and nutrients to all areas of the body and remove waste and carbon dioxide. The heart pumps blood to the capillaries where the blood cells pass through and exchange nutrients and waste; to the lungs where carbon dioxide is exchanged for oxygen; and to the liver and kidneys for waste removal.

The four most *common types of cardiovascular disease* are high blood pressure, coronary heart disease (which includes heart attack), stroke

Muscular System

and rheumatic heart disease. Atherosclerosis occurs when the inner walls of the arteries become narrower due to a buildup of plaque. Blood clots form, obstructing blood flow and causing heart attacks and strokes.

Respiratory system

We breathe with our respiratory system — the intake and the exchange of oxygen and carbon dioxide between our bodies and the environment. Each cell in the body uses oxygen to make

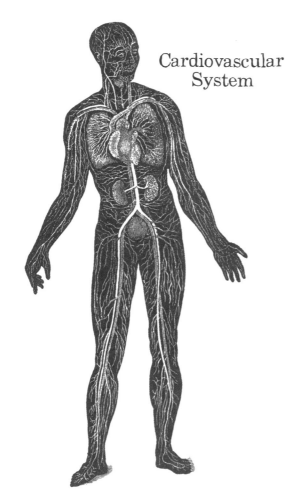

Cardiovascular
System

Nervous system

All of our conscious awareness of the external environment and all of our motor activity to cope with it operate in the nervous system. It is the body's control and communication system and is comprised of several systems that function together. The *central nervous system* is the brain, spinal cord, nerves and sense organs, such as the eye and ear. There are two parts to the *peripheral nervous system — autonomic* and *somatic*. The autonomic nervous system regulates involuntary bodily functions, our internal organs, smooth muscles and glands, our heartbeat. The somatic parts of the peripheral nervous system are the peripheral nerve fibers that send sensory information to the central nervous system and the

energy and produces carbon dioxide as a waste product. Air enters the body through the nose and mouth and travels down the pharynx (throat) to the trachea (windpipe), through the bronchial tubes and into the lungs where it is drawn into numbers of thin-walled air sacs. Here the exchange of oxygen and carbon dioxide in the blood takes place.

Respiratory failure may be caused by lung cancer or tuberculosis. Other disorders include pneumonia, emphysema and asthma.

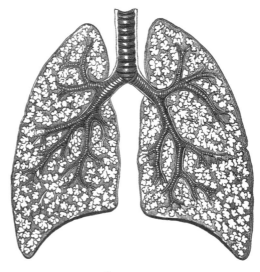

Lungs

motor nerve fibers that activate our skeletal muscles. The nervous system is influenced by the emotions that can affect the rate of the heartbeat.

Diseases of the nervous system that affect the muscles were listed with the muscular aystem. Other *nervous system disorders* include Alzheimer's Disease, brain cancer and tumors, epilepsy and stroke.

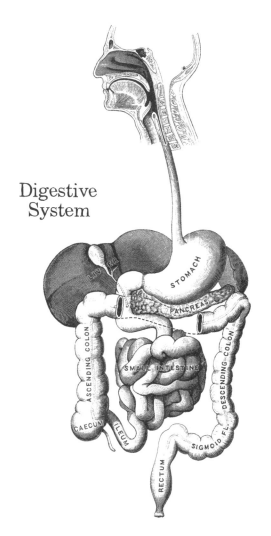

Digestive System

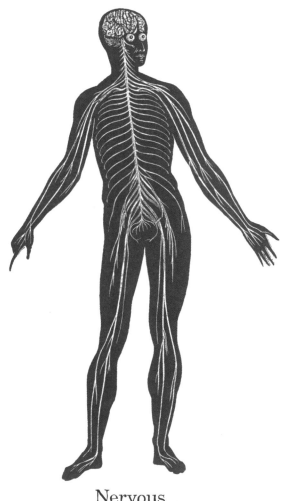

Nervous System

Digestive system

The digestive system, our gastro-intestinal tract, takes in food, digests it to extract energy and nutrients, and expels some wastes. This system has two parts. The *alimentary canal* runs from the mouth, through the pharynx, esophagus, stomach, small and large intestines to the rectum and anus. *Organs and glands*, the teeth, tongue, salivary glands, pancreas, liver and gallbladder, change food mechanically and chemically into a form the body can use.

Common *digestive system diseases* include stomach, liver, pancreatic, colon and other cancers, ulcers, hepatitis, Chrons disease, cirrhosis and acid reflux disease.

Urinary system

The urinary system is responsible for eliminating the body's liquid chemical wastes. Each cell in the body discharges its waste into the bloodstream, which carries the acids, salts and excess fluids for filtering in the kidneys. The waste-filled fluids are collected in the bladder and then excreted as urine.

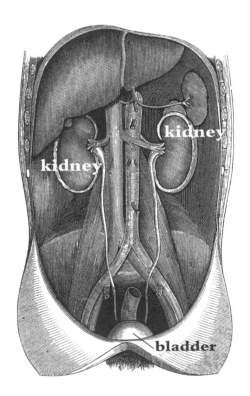

Urinary
System

Generally, we can live well with just one kidney. Only when the amount of functioning kidney tissue is greatly diminished will kidney (renal) failure develop. Depending on the severity of the symptoms, dialysis or kidney transplantation with a suitable donor may occur.

Kidney diseases may be acute or chronic and can lead to renal failure. Chronic kidney disease can be caused by diabetes, high blood pressure, polycystic kidney disease, lupus, improper use of certain medications or kidney stones. Other urinary system disorders include urinary tract infections, prostatitis and cancer of the kidney and bladder.

Reproductive system

The reproductive system consists of the organs that characterize the sexes and allow us to combine genes to create offspring. Male reproductive organs are the penis, scrotum, testes and prostate; the female's, vulva, clitoris, ovaries, cervix, uterus and vagina.

Pregnancy accounts for the largest number of *reproductive system hospitalizations*. Cancer of the prostate, uterus, cervix and ovaries are also common disorders associated with the reproductive system.

Endocrine system

The endocrine system is a system of ductless glands that secretes hormones — chemical messengers that use the bloodstream to circulate throughout the body and regulate its systems. Major glands include: pineal, pituitary, thyroid, thymus, parathyroid, adrenal, pancreas, ovaries and testes.

Common diseases of the endocrine system are diabetes, growth disorders, cancer and thyroid diseases.

Lymphatic system

The lymphatic system defends the body against invasion by disease-causing agents like viruses, bacteria and fungi. Consisting of the bone marrow, spleen, thymus gland, lymph nodes, tonsils, appendix and a few other organs, it is a network of vessels that works with the body's veins to drain fluid from tissues and help defend against infection with infection-fighting cells called *lymphocytes*, produced by stem cells in the bone marrow.

Whenever the lymph system cannot drain fluid from tissues faster than it accumulates, swelling (*lymphedema*) results. Cancers that develop from lymphocytes are *lymphomas*; the two main groups are Hodgkin's disease and non-Hodgkin's lymphoma.

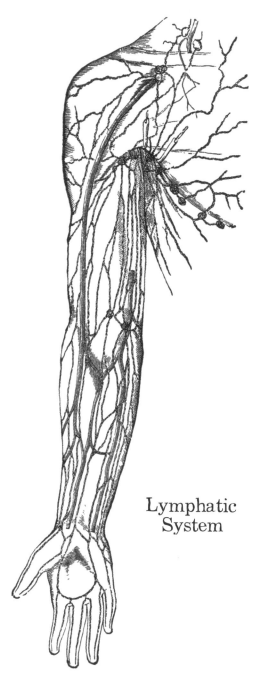

Lymphatic System

Integumentary system

The integumentary system is the largest system of the human body, enclosing and protecting all the body's organs and tissues. Including the skin, hair, nails and cutaneous glands, this ever-changing organ contains specialized cells and structures that maintain the body's temperature, gather information from the environment and play an active role in our immune system. Skin is the body's largest organ.

Skin cancer is the most common type of cancer; the two most frequent types are basal cell carcinoma and squamous cell carcinoma. Melanoma, the third most frequent skin cancer, is a malignancy of the cells that give the skin its color *(melanocytes)*.

Life-Threatening Illnesses — When the Healthy Functioning of Our Bodies Goes Awry

In 1997 when The Creative Center developed its Hospital Artist-In-Residence Program, our artists worked primarily with children and adults who had been diagnosed with cancer. In most hospitals and hospices, however, beds on the oncology floor were also occupied by people living with and being treated for other life-threatening illnesses. Many of our artists developed expertise in working with adults with Parkinson's disease, diabetes, multiple-diagnoses and liver transplants; or with children who were suffering from genetic diseases or rare infections. Building on The Center's overview of the systems of the human body, our artists' training also includes presentations on various life-threatening illnesses.

Overview of human disease

Only two types of diseases affect humans:

- *External* — those caused unnaturally by something outside the body, like a virus, bacteria or toxin.
- *Internal* — those caused naturally when something goes wrong with one or more of the body's systems, an internal "mistake."

There are *external agents,* that clearly cause disease or harm to the body. Some include:

- Bacteria.
- Viruses.
- Parasites.
- Vitamin and mineral deficiencies.
- Toxins.
- Radiation (including natural sunlight and man-made energies).
- Physical damage (accidental or intentional, such as homicide or suicide).

Though some external agents can initiate an internal failing of a body's system, the result is that the body acts improperly — gets into the wrong mode — becomes sick. Some common types of *internal problems* that lead to disease are:

- Inherited genetic defects.
- Cancer.
- Immune-response disorders (including an overactive immune

system and auto-immunity).

- Metabolic disorders.
- Anatomical problems.

Some diseases are a combination of something external triggering an internal response. For instance, no one is sure if cancer is caused by a virus or occurs naturally by the normal process of DNA mutation.

The term *dual diagnoses* is used when a person has more than one disease — HIV-AIDS and tuberculosis, or end-stage cancer and congestive heart failure. People are hospitalized for a variety of serious illnesses; some of the life-threatening illnesses the AIR may see most often are described below.

Cancer
Our bodies are made up of many different types of cells, each of which has a specific purpose. Every minute, ten million cells divide in the human body. Normally, cell division, growth and development occur in an orderly way. Cancer develops from a single cell that has undergone mutations in its DNA and behaves differently. Instead of maturing normally and dying, cancerous cells reproduce without restraint and never mature. Our body has defense mechanisms against cancer cells; when these defenses are ineffective, the result is a diagnosis of cancer.

A single cancerous cell eventually becomes a collection of cells *(tumor)* that invades and destroys surrounding tissue. There are two types of tumors. Cancer cells may be *dispersed* through blood (leukemia) or lymph system (lymphoma) or *solid,* a mass of cancer cells in one organ or part of the body. Cancers are named by what types of cells are overgrowing — by where the tumor occurs.

The two categories of tumors are benign and malignant. A *benign tumor* stays in the tissue in which it arises; it may grow to a size that causes significant problems, but it will not spread to another part of the body. In a *malignant (cancerous) tumor,* cells break off and invade surrounding tissue or travel to other sites in the body where new tumors form. This process of invasion and spread is called *metastasis.*

Cancer is treated by surgery, chemotherapy, radiation therapy and/or biotherapy.

Surgery, the oldest form of cancer treatment, is performed for several reasons: to remove malignant and potentially malignant tissue; to take a sample to determine type, extent and amount of disease; to treat complications of advanced disease; and to reconstruct or restore a patient's appearance or the function of an organ or bodily part after primary surgery. New methods to remove or destroy cancerous tissue are constantly being developed.

Chemotherapy is the treatment of cancer with strong chemicals or drugs, in precisely measured doses, designed to kill rapidly dividing cancer cells. Drugs are given by mouth (orally) or injected into a muscle, a blood vessel (intravenously) or the abdomen or pleural cavity. Entering the blood stream, they are transported throughout the body. In this way chemotherapy can reach cancer cells that are missed by surgery or radiation treatment. Chemotherapeutic drugs may also temporarily damage healthy cells. Side effects depend on the type of drug and dosage and may include:

- Nausea and vomiting.
- Hair loss.
- Fatigue due to the body's inability to produce enough red blood cells; and bruising and bleeding, if the platelets are affected.
- Infection caused by a reduction in the number of white blood cells.

Radiation therapy uses high energy radiation to kill cells, shrink tumors or to keep them from growing. Radiation treatments are often broken down into a series of sessions over time in order to allow damaged normal cells to

repair. Common side effects include:
- Fatigue.
- Loss of appetite and nausea.
- Hair loss.
- Skin damage.

Biotherapy, also known as the use of "biological response modifiers" or "immunotherapy-treatment," is used to augment the body's own resistance and strengthen the immune system. This type of cancer treatment uses naturally occurring substances that are produced by the body's cells (Interleukin-2 and Interferon natural lymphokines) and/or the cells themselves (stimulated immune cells).

Cardiovascular disease

Cardiovascular disease, the leading cause of death for both men and women in the U.S., includes a number of conditions affecting the structures or functions of the heart. These are some of the most common:

- *Coronary artery disease* is atherosclerosis — hardening of the arteries that provide vital oxygen and nutrients to the heart.
- *Heart failure* simply means that the heart is not pumping as well as it should; congestive heart failure causes the blood to back up behind the heart leading to fluid accumulation in the lungs and body.
- *Pericardial disease,* pericarditis,

is an inflammation of the lining that surrounds the heart, usually caused by an infection.

- *Vascular disease* includes any condition that affects the circulatory system including diseases of the arteries and blood flow to the brain.

Treatments for cardiovascular disease depend up the specific form of the disease in each patient, and may include surgery (from heart transplant to bypass), medication and lifestyle changes.

Diabetes

Diabetes is a disorder of metabolism, characterized by elevated blood sugar levels. The food we eat is broken down into glucose, a form of sugar in the blood and the main source of the body's energy. After digestion, glucose passes into the bloodstream. Insulin must be present for glucose to leave the blood and get into our cells. Insulin is produced by the pancreas. In individuals with diabetes, the pancreas produces little or no insulin, or the cells do not respond to the insulin that is produced. Glucose amounts increase in the blood, overflow into the urine and pass out of the body. The diabetic's body is unable to utilize its main source of fuel though the blood contains large amounts. Long-term complications of diabetes can affect almost every part of the body — blindness, heart and blood vessel disease, stroke, kidney failure, amputation and nerve damage.

Some types of diabetes are controlled with lifestyle changes (diet and exercise); others require aggressive monitoring and insulin therapy. In one experimental therapy, cells from a donor's pancreas are transplanted to a person with diabetes.

Parkinson's disease

Parkinson's disease is a degenerative brain disorder affecting one's ability to control movement. In this debilitating and progressive disorder, the cells that produce dopamine, the chemical made in the brain that facilitates electrical transmission between nerve cells, break down causing dopamine levels to drop. Symptoms usually begin in middle to later life with trembling of the lips and hands, loss of facial expression and muscular rigidity. Movements become slow and difficult; dementia and depression are common.

There is no known treatment to stop or reverse the breakdown of these nerve cells. Drugs, and occasionally surgery, can be used to treat the symptoms of the disease.

HIV/AIDS

Human immunodeficiency virus (HIV) is the virus that causes acquired immune deficiency syndrome (AIDS). This virus attacks the immune system, making it difficult for the body to fight infections and cancer. However, having HIV does not mean having AIDS. People with HIV are said to have AIDS when they develop certain infections or cancers, or when the amount of a particular white blood cell (CD4) drops to a low level.

HIV and AIDS cannot be cured, but the disease's progression can be slowed or halted. The most effective treatment for HIV is highly-active anti-retroviral therapy (HAART), a combination of several anti-retroviral medications that decreases the replication of the virus in the body. If HIV is left untreated, it eventually progresses and causes infections, cancer and AIDS.

Life-Threatening Illnesses Common in Children
Leukemia

The most common form of cancer in children, leukemia is cancer of the white blood cells (leukocytes), those cells that help the body fight infections and other diseases. Large numbers of abnormal white blood cells are produced in the bone marrow interfering with the body's production

of red blood cells and platelets. Anemia, bleeding and an increased risk of infection are associated with both acute and chronic leukemias.

With proper treatment the outlook for children diagnosed with leukemia is quite good, with remission rates of up to 90%.

Sickle cell disease

Sickle cell disease, the most commonly occurring genetic disease in the U.S., is a blood disorder found more often in those of African-American descent. Normal round red blood cells move through the body's blood vessels, delivering oxygen. Sickle cell disease causes these cells to be misshapen — they look like sickles or crescent moons. Sickled cells get stuck in blood vessels, blocking blood flow and causing severe pain, anemia and damage to organs, muscles and bones. Children five years and younger face the greatest risk, with death caused by overwhelming infection.

Treatment involves childhood-long monitoring of the child's health and well-being. Education helps parents learn to control symptoms as they arise and to act quickly in an emergency.

Cystic fibrosis

Cystic fibrosis (CF), the most commonly fatal genetic disease in the

U.S. today, is a chronic, progressive condition that primarily affects the respiratory and digestive systems. Due to a gene defect, the mucous the body produces is abnormally thick and sticky. Clogging in the lungs leads to recurring lung and sinus infections as well as difficulty breathing. In the ducts of the pancreas, thick mucous prevents digestive enzymes from reaching the intestines. Those with CF do not absorb nutrients from their food efficiently. CF also damages both the male and female reproductive systems.

The severity of the disease symptoms of CF is directly related to the characteristic effects of the particular mutations that have been inherited by the sufferer. Early diagnosis, improved antibiotic treatment and improved nutritional management enable the majority of children with CF to live well into adulthood.

Asthma
Asthma is a disease of the branches of the windpipe (bronchial tubes), which carry air in and out of the lungs. Bronchial asthma can vary from a mild cough and wheezing to severe respiratory distress that may be fatal. During an attack, three main things happen to make it difficult for air to move freely in the lungs. First, the bands of muscle that surround the

airways tighten, causing them to narrow *(bronchospasm)*. Second, the lining of the airways becomes swollen and inflamed. Finally, the cells that line the airways produce more and thicker mucous. Carbon dioxide is trapped in the lungs, breathing is labored. Many children outgrow their symptoms at puberty; others retain symptoms into their twenties and develop other forms of allergies.

The cause of asthma is unknown and there is no cure. Treatment and control involve avoiding things that trigger an attack, using medications (bronchodilators, anti-inflammatories and other drugs) and carefully monitoring daily symptoms.

Equipment in the Hospital Room
The training the AIR receives from both The Creative Center and the healthcare institution will stress the importance of the artist never touching any of the equipment in a patient's room. If a problem or questionable situation arises, the AIR must call the nurse.

For additional information, see also the glossary of medical terms in Appendix I.

The Portable Studio — Continued!

This appendix continues Chapter 8, *The Portable Studio*. Here you will find information and suggestions in additional media: printmaking, collage and mixed media, modeling clays, book arts, fiber arts and jewelry. There are many other media that artists use successfully in the hospital. Refer to the basics recommended in the chapter and then experiment with what you are interested in. You will discover what works for you and your patients!

Printmaking
Why do printmaking in the hospital?

Printmaking offers the non-artist the opportunity to use a variety of "technical tricks" that, once combined, can produce artwork that is interesting and strong. The processes of various printmaking methods range from simple to complicated, all of which can have a place at the bedside, provided that the inks are water-based. And, since the essence of printmaking is to produce multiples, the patient will be able to produce enough work to give to family, friends, and staff — and still be able to keep one (as well as the original printing plate).

What you need

1. Small tubes of *water-based inks* (Speedball) in a variety of colors, as larger ones can dry out.
2. *Water soluble crayons.*
3. *Thick crayons* for texture rubbings.
4. Commercial *stamp pads.*
5. *Heavyweight cardboard "plates"* no larger than 8" x 10".
6. *Lightweight cardboard, oak tag or card stock* to cut into shapes for collographs.
7. *Styrofoam sheets* for "etching," either purchased from an art supply store or cut from the bottom of vegetable or meat trays.
8. *Plexiglass "plates"* no larger than 8" x 10" for monotypes. (Lightly distress the plate with steel wool to help the ink adhere.)
9. *Brayers (rollers)* no larger than 2".
10. *Japanese barren or wooden spoon* for rubbing.
11. *Brushes* — any good stiff brush

works for painting with ink
on a plexiglass plate.
(Ink is less fluid than paint.)

12. A *metal cookie sheet* that fits
in the box for inking paper.

13. A *metal baking pan* (9" x 12")
for rolling ink.

14. *Old newspaper,* cut to fit into
the cookie sheet.

15. *Textured papers and fabrics,* things
that will make a nice "impression"
(doilies, corrugated papers, lace, cord,
basketweave, corduroy and string).

16. *Small erasers, corks and soft foam*
for carving into for stamp making.

17. *Small pine wood blocks* for making
built-up stamps.

18. *Printmaking tools:* small scissors;
UHU gluesticks or small Elmer's glue;
bamboo skewers or dull pencils (for
incising into Styrofoam); synthetic
sponges in plastic airtight containers
(for holding ink for stamping).

19. *Paper:* soft and absorbent — rice
paper, newsprint, drawing paper,
handmade papers, patterned papers,
printed matter (newspapers, magazine
sheets, hospital menus); construction
paper takes ink well and dries quickly.
(Paper should be pre-cut slightly
larger than the printing plate.)

20. *Water mister.*

21. *Latex-free gloves* for the inking
process.

Getting started

While you are setting up, it's helpful
to show patients some actual prints
or photos that illustrate different
printmaking techniques. With samples,
it is easier to describe the concepts —
reversing the image, positive and
negative, monoprint and ghostprint.
Make sure that your examples are
clear. In addition, the actual plate can
be used to demonstrate the process
— as a dry run through, much like a
flight attendant demonstrating the use
of oxygen masks! It will become very
clear that each time you ink the plate,
you can pull another print.

Collograph
One of the simplest printmaking
techniques at the bedside is the
collograph. Begin a printing plate
by cutting shapes from softer board
(oak tag or cardstock) and glue
them to the cardboard backing. These
shapes can be realistic or abstract and
the design can be simple or complex.
Shapes can glued in a single layer,
or more elaborate collographs can be
constructed by layering many shapes,
such as a Christmas tree that has
round ornaments glued on top. A
border can be created as well, and
textured papers and cloth can be
included. When the image is complete,
lay a thin white paper on top and
make a "rubbing" by working the
side of a soft, dark crayon across it.
The edges of the shapes will appear as
hard edges on the paper. Explain that

this print is a "positive" image, that it is oriented exactly like the plate. Do several rubbings in different colors. Now the patient is ready to ink — another way to make a print from a collograph plate.

Squeeze a small amount of ink in a line in the middle of the baking pan and roll the brayer through it until it is covered with ink. Then, having covered the bottom of the cookie sheet with newspaper, lay the plate in the center of the tray and roll the brayer over it, covering it completely with ink. Have the patient make the first print by placing a paper on top of the plate and rubbing with the barren, spoon or side of fist. Pull off print and put aside. Print at least 3 or 4 more times, rolling more ink onto the plate, if necessary. Water-based ink dries very quickly, so work fast! Explain (and show) how this image is reversed from the image on plate.

Although it is too difficult in the hospital setting to change the color of the ink on the same plate, you can change the look of the print by printing on different colored or patterned papers. Metallic papers can lend a holiday look to any image.

Styrofoam etchings
Styrofoam etchings are another easy way for patients to produce multiples.

Using an incising tool (pencil, nail, toothpick, skewer) have patient draw on the styrofoam plate, using enough pressure to make a clear indentation. Point out that the "line" they create will retain the color of the paper, and the raised sections (non-incised) will pick up the ink. Remind them that because this will print in the reverse (as a mirror image), any words must be written backwards (even individual letters must be flipped!). Apply the ink in the same manner as in collograph printing, taking care not to ink heavily (the indentations should not fill with ink). Lay a clean sheet of paper, colored or white, on top of the Styrofoam, and use hand pressure (or the back of a wooden spoon) to rub, transferring the image to the paper. Pull off and set aside to dry. When dry, inked prints may be trimmed and mounted on notecards made from cardstock.

Stamping
Another form of printmaking to try is *stamping*. Stamps can be created by incising, or building. For incised stamps, use carving tools to create grooves in corks or soft erasers. For handmade stamps, ask patients to cut shapes from soft foam or cardboard (like collographs) and glue them to small pine blocks. Cord or string can also be glued to wood blocks to make designs that can be inked by pressing them onto sponges that have been

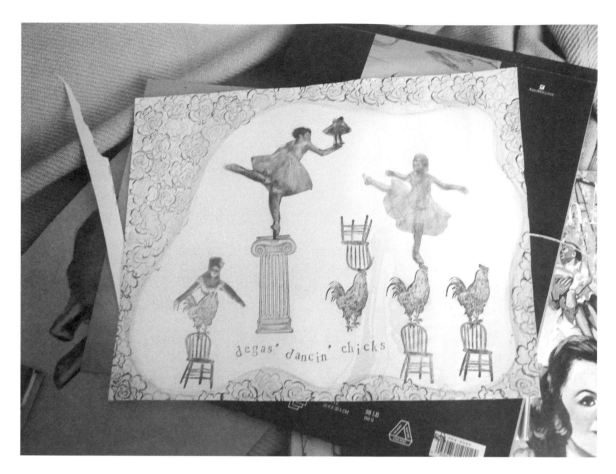

covered in ink or paint, or commercial stamp pads. Commercial rubber stamps are fun, too, and a complete alphabet is also handy.

Monotypes
Monotypes, which means "one print," are created by painting on a plexiglass plate using water-based inks or water-soluable crayons. When you are satisfied with image on the painted plate, you can transfer it to a piece of paper. Lay the paper on top of the plate and rub with your hands, a spoon or a Japanese barren. If the ink appears to have dried, use a water mister on the paper to reactivate it for printing. When the print is "pulled,"

most of the image will have transferred to the paper, in the reverse. Sometimes there is enough ink left on the plate to pull a second, much lighter print — the "ghost." When it dries, the ghost can be used as a starting point or "underpainting" for another drawing or painting.

Collage and Mixed Media
Why do collage in the hospital?
Many AIRs (and patients) find that collage and mixed media are the most accessible art forms, and the easiest for the AIR to "sell." Many patients find comfort in found images (much less threatening than a blank paper), and will spend lots of time associating with

and talking about them before beginning to make art. Cutting and gluing are familiar and easy skills — all keys to success.

The hospital environment is typically devoid of color and texture and collage provides both. Selection, placement and manipulation of a pre-existing image (and often text) returns the power of decision making to patients who may have lost that ability upon entering the hospital. The abundant nature of collage, the "more than you could ever use" amount of materials that an AIR provides to the patient in the bed is the true gift of this medium.

What you need
1. A *tray with many compartments* to hold collage materials, preferably with a snaptight lid.
2. *Portable CD case* with plastic sleeves to hold text and images pre-cut from newspapers and magazines, organized by subject.
3. *Gallon-size Ziploc bags* filled with pre-cut images organized by color, subject, shape.
4. *Papers:* patterned, textured, unusual, metallic, gift wrap (seasonal and celebratory), Asian, handmade, painted, maps, comics, menus — anything you can find!
5. *Collage materials:* small natural objects (shells, leaves, pressed flowers, twigs, feathers), decorative ribbons, buttons, sequins, beads, anything shiny or glitzy.
6. *Magazines:* nature, travel, art, food — anything that might be of interest to the patient.
7. *Surfaces:* plain cardboard, matboard, cigar boxes, small papier mache boxes, pre-cut small mats to decorate as picture frames.
8. UHU or Prang *glue sticks* for paper work, Elmer's glue for small lightweight objects, Tacky glue for heavier objects.
9. *Cutting tools:* small, sharp scissors for intricate cutting, Fiskar's fancy-edged scissors for decorative cutting, hole punchers in various shapes.
10. Alphabet and other *rubber stamps and stamp pad.*

Getting started
Many AIRs describe collage to the patients they work with as simply "a chance to decorate." Decoration is something everyone can understand, and when presented with a wide array of materials, most people will happily begin. Occasionally, a patient must be coaxed to "do a little more," with the AIR making suggestions. Depending on the backing surface, patients can create a functional item (a frame, box or card) or can make an "art collage" inspired by the Dada collagists, Max Ernst and Hannah Höch. The collage may be as simple as a collection of things the patient likes.

The absurdity and bizarreness of altered images can have a lighthearted or powerful theme, depending on the types of images as well as the references you used for inspiration. Reproductions of African-American artist Romare Bearden's well-known collage, *The Street*, or any of his works about his boyhood will resonate with patients. Combining collage with drawing and painting, Bearden often reconstructed his past, as well as historical events. Patients can be encouraged to think about an event that they would like to depict. One AIR brings photocopied enlargements of famous people (movie stars, government officials, historical characters) and places (natural settings like the Grand Canyon, as well as architectural wonders such as the Colosseum, the Eiffel Tower and the Empire State Building) that can be changed radically and comically with the myriad of collage elements. Photocopying multiples of an image to present to patients can also have a powerful effect in a collage — fifty cows marching across Fifth Avenue, or twenty rubber boots climbing the Rocky Mountains.

Using a patient's drawing as the background, collage elements can be added to create a more intricate and imaginative scene. Likewise, old maps, menus, advertisements, advertising flyers and "retired" game boards can be re-appropriated through collage. One patient re-imagined "Monoply," using elements of his own life as both the board and the playing cards!

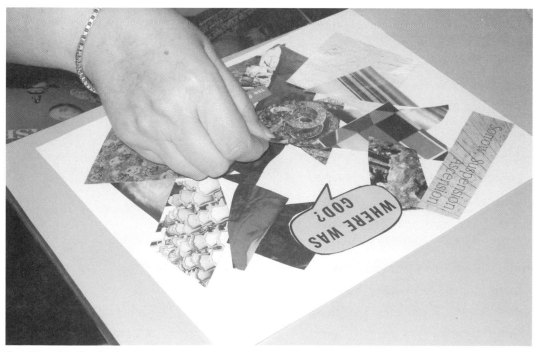

Modeling Clays
Why use modeling clays in the hospital?

Although raw clay is simply too messy to use at the bedside, there are modeling materials available that are wonderfully suited to this pliable and elastic artform. The sheer pleasure in squeezing a ball of plasticene or Model Magic is evident — many patients report a "sense memory" of molding dough as children, while others laugh gleefully as the excess shoots out from between their fingers. The hospital room offers little in the way of tactile pleasures — hard, cool edges and scratchy, stiff fabric. Modeling doughs are the perfect antidote — soft, warm and impressionable. Whether you choose to offer a dough that can be air-dried (Play-Doh, Model Magic), hardens in the oven (Sculpey, Fimo), or one that never hardens (plasticene, plastilina), the experience of "transforming" a lump of clay is "transformative!"

Most adult patients will tell you that they have never worked with "clay" (we will call all modeling materials "clay") or they only worked with it in the art room at school when they were children. However, that doesn't prevent them from immediately grasping it and squeezing, pulling and poking! Like drawing, modeling in clay often begins exactly where your patient left off as a child — for many, it's a three-ball snowman, or little bowl or volcano, while others squeeze and pound, squeeze and pound. And, of course, there is always the ever-popular snake!

What you need

1. A *variety of clays (modeling materials):* Crayola's Model Magic, both white and colors, a lightweight, delightful material that can be sculpted to fine detail and air-dried or stored in airtight containers or bags (buy small 4oz. packages, not the tub which dries out quickly); Play-Doh; Sculpey and Fimo polymer clays (remain pliable at room temperature but can be baked to harden); soft plasticene or plastilina (natural clay mixed with oil — a non-hardening, clean clay which comes in different degrees of hardness).

2. *Clay tools:* small rolling pins, orange sticks, toothpicks, cookie cutters, plastic knives, nylon filament (for making clean cuts in the dough), plastic drinking straws (to mold beads around).

3. *Jewelry findings:* clasps, cords, jump rings and pin backs for transforming beads into jewelry.

Getting started

Arrive in a patient's room with a ball of modeling clay in your hand — divide it in two and place a piece directly into the hand of the patient — irresistible! While you are arranging the work surface and the "sculpting tools," let the patient squeeze, poke, pull and roll — these things happen quite naturally. It is the "playing" that is absorbing. The ability to create and squash, create and squash, can be very freeing because there is no permanent "record" of the creation. Patients can be as absurd as they want — no holds barred!

Reluctant patients might respond to a clay "game." Begin by presenting a lump of clay that you, the AIR, do something to. Then it's the patient's turn — add, subtract, twist, pull, stretch. Use some of the clay tools to alter the clay.

Modeling clay can be used in a game much like "Pictionary." Have a prepared deck of cards with suggestions written on each: "Make a cat," "Make a human (or android),"

"Use three colors to make your favorite food." Model Magic, in particular, is perfect for shaping finger puppets — particularly helpful when there are young visitors or patients. These can be left to dry and may be colored later with paints or markers.

Fimo and Sculpey are fabulous for making beads, pendants and brooches. Both are polymer clays which must be baked in the home oven, either by the AIR if the patient is long-term, or sent home with the patient or family (take-out food containers with snap-tight lids make handy transportation). Be sure you leave the proper jewelry findings to complete the project. Polymer clay aficionados have extensive websites filled with great ideas. Metallic and iridescent clays are a sure hit in the bland hospital environment — you'll probably have many staff members lining up to work with you as well!

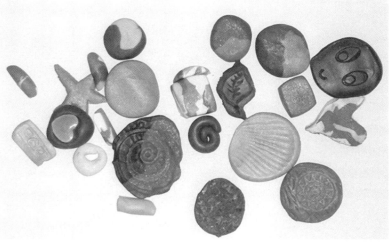

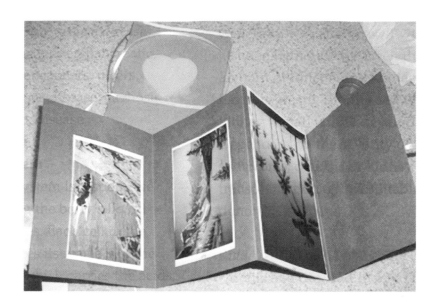

Book Arts
Why create artist books in the hospital?

Small, simple artist books can be made easily at the bedside — the pages filled or left blank for another time. A small blank book can provide an intimate experience for the patient, rich with possibilities of endless variations that are dependent only on the vision. Even the simplest book forms, no matter how humble or easily crafted, can have depth beyond what the materials may suggest. A book can house thoughts or dreams. It can hold memories or a tribute to a special person. It can become a diary, or a record of time spent (in the hospital or on a vacation). It can keep recipes, photographs, addresses or "To Do" lists. A book can hold autographs, interesting newspaper clippings or artwork. Patients may tell a story in a book or ask friends to contribute one. There are books that seem made for holding wishes, and others that can hold information. With five or six book forms, an AIR can offer patients the opportunity to create something that may be meaningful and will last for a long time.

What you need

1. *Paper:* 8½" x 11" white and colored paper, cardstock, index cards, small envelopes, decorative papers, origami patterned papers.

2. *Binding materials:* hole punch, twine, rubber bands, yarn, small twigs, thin ribbon, embroidery thread.

3. *Sharp scissors.*

4. *Art knife* (for AIR use only).

5. *Bone folder or letter opener* for making sharp folds.

6. *Writing tools:* fine point markers, gel pens, metallic pens, glitter pens,

India ink pen stix, crayons, press-on letters, alphabet rubber stamps, "glow-in-the-dark" pens, colored pencils.

7. UHU or Prang *gluesticks*.
8. *Magazines* for collage.

Getting started

It's a good idea to make a variety of sample book forms (both blank and filled) using beautiful papers for patients to choose from and to photocopy directions for each type to leave with them. Some AIRs prepare individual kits in Ziploc bags that include both materials and directions.

There are countless websites and books about making artist books. Directions for some of the easier book forms can be found by typing in the name of the more popular book types: stick and rubber band book, tunnel book, wish scroll, "hotdog book," index card book and envelope book.

Since many simple book forms take so little time, be prepared to make a few types or bring supplies for filling the pages. Small books lend themselves to collage, stamping, illuminated lettering, embellished borders, drawings and photographs. Stencils and templates, as well as rubber stamps and stickers can personalize a book quickly and easily. At the patient's direction, AIRs can use extra-sharp art knives and cutting mats to shape pages intricately or create pop-up designs.

I worked for many weeks with only one of the patients in a double room. The woman in the other bed was always surrounded by her daughters, at least seven or eight of them, ranging in age from ten to thirty. One day, as I was walking out, she called to me, "Hey, how about me?" Her daughters parted and pulled over a chair for me. "I want you should write how I cook the food."

I quickly pulled out some large index cards and began to take dictation in broken English and idiomatic Yiddish, which sent her daughters into fits of laughter. As I finished each recipe, I would give it to one of "the girls" along with a handful of colored pencils. They decorated the borders, as well as every bit of blank space, with pictures of the food they grew up with — gefilte fish, matzoh ball soup, noodle kugel. We worked for three weeks on the cookbook, which I bound simply by punching holes and threading them with cord. I've always wondered which one of the daughters would keep it — and if they ever thought to make photocopies.

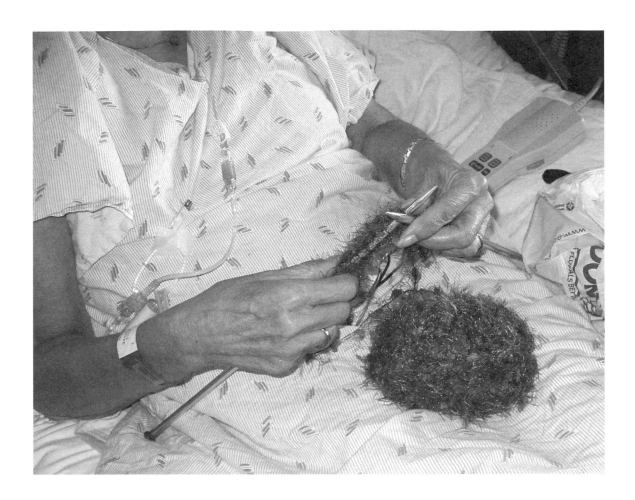

Fiber Arts
Why sew (knit, crochet, embroider, weave) in the hospital?

Illness can take away a lot of things from a patient — peace of mind, the ability to look forward, a sense of well being. As one cancer patient put it, "Each morning, I would open my eyes and the word CANCER would magically appear in big block letters. I could see through it, like a window screen, but it was always there, sometimes faintly, but always present." The omnipresent fear that a patient must cope with every day, combined with lots of time for "what if?" "what's next?" and

"what's happening to me?" can be as debilitating as the illness itself. Knitting, and all the other fiber arts, settle a lot of that "noise" because counting stitches, reading patterns, threading needles, balling yarn and knotting threads require actions that are both repetitive and soothing. And the tactile nature of cloth and yarn is an age-old soother — remember your security blanket?

Sometimes it's not the patient in the bed who needs soothing, but the family members who have spent many hours or even days at the bedside. Long periods of quiet boredom can raise anxiety levels sky high, particularly when a patient is in pain or non-communicative.

Fiber projects are "clean" projects in the hospital, easily started, easily ended. They can be continued after the AIR leaves the room or after the patient leaves the hospital. Their familiar nature makes it easy for patients to say, "yes," and are often talking points when healthcare staff enters the room. (Staff at one NYC hospital have formed a knitting circle for both men and women.) Everyone, it seems, has a mother, grandmother or aunt who did some form of fiber arts in their childhood — another positive association.

What you need

Materials: Outfit the portable fiber studio with at least three or four complete set-ups for a variety of projects.

Knitting

1. *Knitting needles:* at least three pair, No. 8 or larger, one for demonstration purposes, and the other two for the patient and visitors.

2. *Yarns:* bright colors make instruction easier; basic acrylic yarn is fine for teaching purposes; soft yarns in luscious colors bring a sense of luxury to the hospital room. (Patients may just want to touch angora and mohair.)

3. Small *scissors.*

4. *Pre-printed directions* for simple projects, as well as websites for instruction at home.

5. Large *Ziploc bags* for holding work.

6. *Permanent marker* for writing names on bag.

Crochet

1. *Crochet hooks:* medium size or larger.

2. Same as above, oriented toward simple crochet projects.

Embroidery and Crewel

1. *Needles:* look for needles specifically made for embroidery or crewel; in the hospital, large eyes and blunted tips work best.

2. *Floss and yarn:* pre-cut a rainbow of colors into workable lengths, making sure there is enough of each color to complete the project.

3. *Cloth:* preprinted designs on muslin are inexpensive and readily available, but many AIRs prefer for the patient to design their own patterns. Use graph paper (for cross-stitch designs) or tracing and transfer paper (like carbon paper) that is specifically made for cloth.

4. *Plastic mesh,* available in craft stores, is very easy to sew and can be cut into bookmark or other shapes for decoration.

5. Small *scissors.*

6. Large *Ziploc bags* for holding work.

7. *Permanent marker* for labeling bag.

Weaving

1. *Looms:* small looms can be made easily from stiff board (heavyweight cardboard or Masonite) that is notched and pre-strung with warp. You can purchase pre-cut looms from many craft sources. Tablet weaving is a more complex form of weaving that produces beautiful, usable results: belts, headbands, bookmarks. A good website with links to various instructional sites is: *www.42explore.com/weave.htm.*

2. *Yarns:* weaving is a perfect way to use up small bits of yarn. Yarn stores and friends are great resources for scraps and tidbits. Jersey cotton (from T-shirts) cut into narrow strips work well by themselves (think rag rug) or in combination with yarns. Thicker yarn is easier to work with and makes completion quicker. Be sure to include some luxurious yarns and ribbons — glitzy is good!

3. *Other fibers:* weavings can be created using all natural materials, or they can be used in combination with commercial yarns. Feathers, reeds, hemp, straw, grasses and weeds bring the natural world into the antiseptic hospital environment.

Getting started

Because so many fiber arts are familiar to people there is a good chance that the patient will be receptive to at least one. Prepackaged kits (made by the AIR) are handy and can be left with a patient or family member to work on later. Have some aspects of the work done already: pre-thread embroidery needles, have yarn already cast on the knitting needles, pre-string the looms. Make sure to include printed instructions in each kit.

Mrs. Alvarado speaks very little English but immediately responds to the embroideries. She chooses her colors and moves back and forth to her husband's bedside, speaking to his suffering. Then she comes back to sit beside me and continues her sewing. This pattern repeats itself as I roll enough yarn for her. As I leave the room she says, "God bless you."

Jewelry
Why make jewelry in the hospital?

Beautiful beads, shiny findings, silken cords in rainbow colors — how better to brighten up a patient wearing a hospital gown? By offering a wide array of colorful and lustrous objects the AIR is perceived by patients, family members and staff as a "gift-giver." The bracelet or necklace that is made by the patient is often "re-gifted" to family or staff, giving the patient an experience that is normalizing and generous.

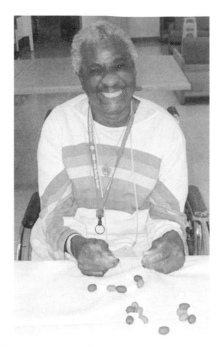

What you need

1. A *felt cloth* cut to fit on top of lid. (The felt keeps the beads from rolling.)
2. *Paper plates* for holding beads.
3. A *large amount of beads* of all types: wood, glass, metal, plastic, alphabet, natural. (Include various pendants and spacers to create a real stand-out.) Organize in divided boxes or small Ziploc bags. Beads and all kinds of supplies can be purchased from: *www.firemountaingems.com.*
4. *Findings, etc.:* monofiliment, jewelry elastic, silk cording, earring wires, pin backs (and glue); clasps, claws and other closings; jump rings.
5. *Tools:* needle-nosed pliers, scissors.
6. Optional: *bead boards* which are grooved for laying out the design.

Getting started

AIRs can enter patient rooms wearing some of their own creations — a living, breathing "sample sale!" Arms loaded with bracelets, the AIR should have no trouble getting positive responses. One AIR removes an item of jewelry from her arm or neck and puts it right on the patient — the first gift!

Placing the lapboard across the patient, lay out your wares like a traveling salesperson. Although the patient will obviously work with a very small amount of beads the experience of choosing a few from so many is half the fun! The only other decision-making he or she will have that day will probably be choosing tomorrow's lunch!

Be prepared to do some, if not all, of the finishing work. Knotting and crimping (squeezing the metal closings) may be too difficult for the patient right now. However, you should demonstrate what you're doing so patients can learn how to do it themselves.

Beading and other forms of jewelry making are equally popular with staff. Workshops for nurses and other healthcare workers can be set up easily, either with instruction or with a more casual "drop-in" approach during lunch hours. One cancer center now has a "bead station" set up permanently in the nurses' lounge, stocked by donations.

Recommended Resources

The following contains a selection of websites, books, magazines, art materials, art supply sources and organizations. This list is not meant to be inclusive but to share some of those we have found most helpful.

Art Websites

www.makingbooks.com*:* simple, clear directions for a number of book designs including "hot dog book," "stick and elastic book," "Ethiopian wish scrolls" and "step books."

www.artistbooks.com*:* a source for books that really raises the bar on the possibilities for artist books; beautiful examples of many book forms; projects; workshop announcements around the U.S.

www.crayola.com*:* designed in three sections — children, parents and educators. Click on "Educators" and follow the link to "Crayola Dream Makers" — a comprehensive resource guide and unique art project ideas.

www.art21.org*:* an expansion of the PBS television series offering lots of information about art — from art historical information to artist bios to projects based on existing artwork —

all of which are easily adaptable to AIR work.

www.whitney.org*:* the official website for The Whitney Museum of American Art in New York City with two links that are especially helpful to AIRs — "Artport" and "Learning." Both are filled with amazing resources and ideas based on contemporary culture.

www.moma.org*:* the Museum of Modern Art's amazing on-line collection of art, as well as links to new exhibits and their permanent collection.

www.metmuseum.org*:* official website for The Metropolitan Museum of Art in NYC with lots of interesting information. Click on "Explore and Learn" for ideas and projects and visit their on-line museum.

www.sculpey.com*:* a good resource for innovative uses of polymer clay, especially sings the praises of Sculpey.

www.polymercafe.com*:* another site for polymer clay fanatics.

www.youthlearn.org*:* great website for an in-depth explanation of inquiry-based questioning to use for art appreciation conversations with patients or caregivers. Click on the "Learn" link and go to "The Art of the Question."

www.42explore.com/weave.htm: lots of information about weaving with links to many other sites.

Magazines

Cloth Paper Scissors, Quilting Arts. Focused on fiber arts and collage work, including mixed media, assemblage, altered books, art dolls, visual art journals, rubber stamping, creative embroidery and book arts.

School Arts, Davis Publications. Aimed at school art teachers, this magazine features many adaptable projects and processes for work with children and adults.

Somerset Studio Magazine*, Stampington and Co. This magazine features paper arts, book arts, art stamping and calligraphy.

Books for Making Art with Children and Adults

Peot, Margaret. **Make Your Mark: Explore Your Creativity and Discover Your Inner Artist.** San Francisco: Chronicle Books LLC, 2004. This book, filled with art techniques ranging from stenciling to rubbings and everything in between, offers a warm, engaging and encouraging voice, helpful tips and clear explanations, all illustrated with actual techniques. Even if you think you know every technique, you're sure to discover something new here.

Rollins, Judy and L. Lawrence Riccio. **Art is the heART: An Arts-in-Healthcare Program for Children and Families in Home and Hospice Care.** Washington, DC: WVSA arts connection, 2001.
This book describes WVSA arts connection's ART is the heART program and provides the reader with the detailed information needed to develop, implement, and evaluate a home-based arts program for children who are ill or dying or children who have a family member who is dying.

Silberstein-Storfer, Muriel. **Doing Art Together.** New York: Harry Abrams, revised, 1997.
Based on the methods used in the renowned parent-child workshops at the Metropolitan Museum of Art, this book presents a hands-on art course that demystifies the artmaking process with understandable step-by-step projects. Shows how to lead others in discovering the natural ways of working with paint, paper and clay — perfect for working with patients!

Watt, Fiona, Antonia Miller, Nonn Figg. **The Usborne Book of Art Projects.** Tulsa, OK: EDC Publishing/Usborne Books, 2004.
Watt, Fiona; Antonia Miller, Katrina Fearn, Natacha Goransky, Vici Leyhane, Howard Allman.

The Usborne Book of Art Skills.
Tulsa, OK: EDC Publishing/Usborne
Books, 2003.
Both provide the AIR with clear and
imaginative skills-based and project-
based art that is easily adaptable to
the hospital setting.

Hellmuth, Claudine. **Collage
Discovery Workshop: Beyond
the Unexpected.** Cincinnati:
North Light Books, 2005.
Packed with original ideas and
artwork, offering some unique
processes that include work with
photos, lettering and hand-drawn
elements on surfaces canvas, fabric,
altered books, paper. Many examples.

Michael, Karen. **The Complete Guide
to Altered Imagery: Mixed Media
Techniques for Collage, Altered
Books, Artists Journals and More.**
Gloucester, MA: Rockport, 2005.
A beautiful book, filled with ideas for
altering real photographs and images
from other sources including magazines
and postage stamps. Many techniques,
from very simple (scratching into
photos) to more elaborate (image
transfer processes) are explained and
illustrated.

Schuman, Jo Miles. **Art From Many
Hands: Multicultural Art Projects.**
Worcester, MA: Davis, 2003.
Both art projects and their cultural
references using easily understood
directions. Ethnic crafts, from Chinese

calligraphy to Pueblo pottery, with
photos of the "authentic" and the
student-made "interpretation."

Terzian, Alexandra. **The Kids'
Multicultural Art Book: Art &
Craft Experiences from Around
the World.** Nashville, TN:
Williamson, 1993.
Very simple projects using household
materials that produce artwork with a
"global spin." Perfect for use with kids
both at the bedside and in groups.

Books of General Interest to Arts in Healthcare Artists

Albom, Mitch. **Tuesdays with Morrie:
An Old Man, a Young Man, and
Life's Greatest Lesson.** New York:
Broadway, 2002.
The author shares weekly discussions
with his terminally ill former
professor, Morrie Schwartz, who
teaches us about living life until
the very end.

Barthes, Roland. **Camera Lucida:
Reflections on Photography.**
New York: Hill and Wang, 1982.
Barthes was a French philosopher
and cultural critic. When his mother,
with whom he had lived his entire
life, dies, he turns to photographs of
her in hopes of glimpsing again her
"essence." He ponders what a photo
is and means to the photographer,
subject and viewer — what we hope
to see and what is really there. Will
change how you look at photographs.

Lipson, Juliene G., Suzanne L. Dibble, Pamela A. Minarik, Eds. **Culture and Nursing Care: A Pocket Guide.** San Francisco: UCSF Nursing Press, 1996. From American Indians to West Indians, this book provides guidelines to the similarities and differences within and among people, as a first step to providing individualized care.

May, Rollo. **Courage to Create.** New York: W.W. Norton and Company, 1994. May, a psychoanalyst, postulates that logic and science derives from art — not the other way around. He encourages readers to discover their creative impulses, offering new possibilities for achievement.

Art Materials Mail Order Sources

Classroom Direct, 1-800-248-9171
www.classroomdirect.com

Sax Arts & Crafts, 1-800-558-6696
www.saxarts.com

Economy Handicrafts, 1-800-216-1601
www.economyhandicrafts.com

Dick Blick Art, 1-800-828-4548
www.dickblick.com

Fire Mountain Beads, 1-800-423-2319
www.firemountaingems.com

Sunshine Crafts, 1-800-729-2878
www.sunshinecrafts.com

Herrschners Yarn, 1-800-441-0838
www.herrschners.com

Pearl Art Supply, 1-800-451-7327
www.pearlpaint.com

Items We Have Used and Liked:

"Sterilite 10-Gallon Tote Box"
#69703-00, 20.5"l x 14.1"w x 12.5"h

Glues
UHU and Prang, gluesticks, for paper
Tacky glue, for heavier objects
Elmer's glue, for lightweight objects

Clays
Crayola Model Magic (4 oz. packages)
Play-Doh
Sculpey and Fimo (polymer)

Pan watercolors
Yarka, Prang

Markers, pencils, pastels, etc.
Crayola Magic Markers (not washable)
Sakura Cray-Pas oil pastels (box of 16)
Prismacolor watercolor pencils
Crayola crayons (box of 64)
Acquarelle watercolor crayons
Sharpie markers, India ink pen stix

Miscellaneous
Styrofoam sheets
Speedball water-based printing inks
Fiskar's fancy-edged scissors
Dr. Marten's inks
Pink Pearl or kneaded eraser

Organizations

Art & Creative Materials Institute
P. O. Box 479
Hanson, MA 02341-0479
www.acminet.org

Society for the Arts in Healthcare
2437 15th St. NW
Washington, DC 20009
202-299-9770
mail@thesah.org, www.thesah.org

Concepts:
Arts in Healthcare

Arts in Healthcare Concepts

In the field of Arts in Healthcare (AIH), there exist several dichotomies. Many in our field seem to favor one side strongly while the more clinical members of the healthcare community are more partial to the other. It is helpful to the AIR to be aware of the ways these concepts are understood and explained by many AIH practitioners.

Cure/Heal

Cure is a method or course of medical treatment used to regain health. *Heal* is often used to refer to the restoring of one's spirit and emotional well-being, independent of one's physical health.

Medicine cures the body.
Art heals the spirit.

Few AIH practitioners claim that they can cure disease, but what the arts can do is help patients access their emotions and essential creativity, sometimes in spite of the progress of their disease.

Interdisciplinary/Multidisciplinary

In our highly specialized medical environment, an *interdisciplinary* approach means working toward a more integrated way of working — bridging the disciplines — communicating and collaborating across specialties. *Multidisciplinary*, in medicine, is a term used to describe an approach in which a number of professionals who are experts at different specialties are brought together to form a treatment team.

An AIR may begin working at a hospital in a multidisciplinary way. But ideally, as time passes and the medical staff becomes acquainted with the benefits of incorporating the arts, the AIR, and all he has to offer, will become integrated into the patients' lives and the fabric of the healthcare institution.

Participation/Observation

Participation is the act of taking part or engaging in an activity; whereas *observation* is a more passive pastime of noting or taking into account.

An arts program in a healthcare setting can offer aspects of both kinds of experiences. Original artworks hung on hospital walls

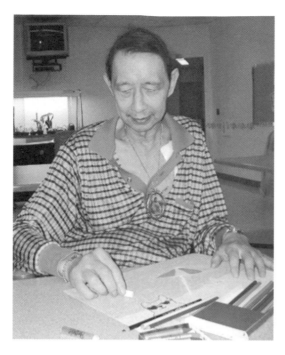

offer an observational experience. An AIR making art with a patient is more active and relational, more stimulating and creative.

Process/Product

Process is a series of actions, changes or functions bringing about a result or *"product."*

Process allows one to gain an understanding or acceptance of one's emotional or psychological being. Making art with an AIR is much more about giving the patient a way to engage his or her creativity. There is little expectation of a fine-art level of finished product. As with "participation" above, successful artmaking in the hospital is about experiencing the activity — involving the patient or caregiver — rather than producing a predetermined result.

Spirituality/Religion

Spirituality encompasses a person's sense of meaning and purpose in life, and can also include a relationship to a higher power or energy that gives life meaning. *Religion* is a specific system of beliefs concerning the sacred, supernatural or divine, and the moral codes, practices, rituals, values and institutions associated with such beliefs.

The hospital is an emotionally charged environment and the AIR may encounter patients who are thinking about or questioning their personal spirituality and religious beliefs. Patients, caregivers, AIRs — anyone — may search for the spiritual, independent of a religious context. Some feel that artmaking offers a spiritual experience.

Therapeutic/Therapy

Therapeutic refers to a general having or exhibiting powers conducive to good health of body or mind; whereas *therapy* is a systematic application of remedies to effect good physical and mental health.

AIRs often state that artmaking is therapeutic — participating in the process is distracting; accessing one's creative resources may be healing. Since artists are not acting as, nor are they trained to be, therapists, what an AIR does is not therapy.

Glossary:
Arts in Healthcare

Acute: transient, of short duration

Allopathic medicine: refers to the type of medicine practiced by MDs and DOs, conventional medicine

Alternative medicine: any of various complete systems of theory and practice for healing or treating disease that are based on alternative traditions or practices and used *in place of* conventional medicine; alternative medical systems include chiropractic, homeopathy, naturopathy and acupuncture

Anxiety: an overwhelming sense of apprehension and fear often marked by physiological signs (such as sweating, tension, and increased pulse), by doubt concerning the reality and nature of the threat, and by self-doubt about one's capacity to cope with it

Aphasia: loss or impairment of the power to use and/or comprehend words, usually resulting from brain damage

Artist: a person skilled in creative activity, such as painting, sculpture, writing, dance, music, etc.

Artist-In-Residence: an artist who is trained to provide artistic engagements to patients and caregivers in hospitals, hospices and other healthcare settings

(the) Arts: the conscious use of skill and creative imagination in visual, literary and performing media

Art therapist: one who is licensed to practice art therapy

Art therapy: psychotherapy that incorporates the production of visual art, such as painting or sculpture, in order to understand and express one's feelings

Benign tumor: an abnormal, localized growth that is not cancerous and does not spread to other areas of the body

Bereavement: the period after a loss during which grief is experienced and mourning occurs

Bone marrow transplant (BMT): a procedure in which bone marrow that is diseased is replaced with healthy bone marrow (a BMT is used to treat malignancies, certain forms of anemia, and immune deficiencies)

Cachectic: physical wasting with loss of weight and muscle mass due to disease

Caregiver: anyone who provides assistance and care to someone in need, often over a long period of time — not only medical, nursing and physical help, but also companionship

Chapbook: a small book containing ballads, poems, tales or tracts

Character disorders: also called personality disorders, are characterized by a persistent pattern of maladaptive behaviors that bring a person repeated conflict and friction with his or her social and occupational environment; these individuals may be narcissistic, obsessive compulsive, sociopathic, avoidant, dependent, etc.

Chemotherapy: the use of chemical agents in the treatment or control of disease

Child life specialist: guided by the philosophy of "family-centered care," supports the psychosocial development of children who are hospitalized, provides them with developmentally appropriate activities that help them and their families adjust to illness and hospitalization

Chronic: long-lasting

Complementary medicine: a method of healthcare that combines the therapies and philosophies both of conventional medicine and alternative medicine, such as using music to help lessen a patient's discomfort following surgery

Death: has occurred when a person's heart no longer beats and there are no signs of breathing; the end of life

Depression (clinical): a state of sadness, dejection and hopelessness that has advanced to the point of being disruptive to an individual's social functioning and/or activities of daily living; a brain disorder that affects the whole body

Depression (reactive): depression precipitated by something intensely sad or distressing

Dyspnea: difficulty in breathing, often associated with lung or heart disease and resulting in shortness of breath

Healthcare: efforts made to maintain or restore health, especially by trained and licensed professionals

Health Insurance Portability and Accountability Act (HIPAA): a federal law that requires a patient's permission to disclose or use any medical information

Holistic medicine: an approach to medical care that promotes wellness and emphasizes all aspects of a person's health — physical, social, psychological, economic, cultural

Hospice care: a type of palliative care in which the patient agrees to forgo curative and life-sustaining treatments; the emphasis is control of pain and discomfort

Hospital: an institution where the sick or injured are given medical and/or surgical care

In-patient: one who stays overnight or longer for treatment in a hospital

Integrative medicine: collaboration of conventional and alternative therapies working together to help the patient

Intravenous (IV): into a vein, for example intravenous (IV) antibiotics are a solution containing antibiotics that is administered directly into the venous circulation via a syringe or intravenous catheter (tube)

Joint Commission on Accreditation of Healthcare Organizations (JCAHO): an independent, not-for-profit organization, established more than 50 years ago, it sets the standards by which healthcare quality is measured in America and around the world. JCAHO recognizes that the needs of patients extend beyond purely physical care to include the mind and spirit.

Leukemia: cancer of the blood forming tissues (bone marrow,

lymph nodes, spleen) characterized by overproduction of abnormal, immature, white blood cells

Lymph: a clear fluid collected by the lymph system that helps the body defend against infection

Lymphedema: a condition of localized swelling (fluid retention) caused by a compromised lymph system

Lymphoma: a cancer of the lymph glands or lymphatic system

Magnetic Resonance Imaging (MRI): a diagnostic process that provides X-ray-like pictures using magnetic fields not radiation

Malignant tumor: a tumor made up of the type of cancer cells that can spread to other parts of the body

Metastasis: the spread of cancer from its primary site to other places in the body

Narcotics: a substance that, in moderate doses, relieves pain, dulls the senses, and induces profound sleep; most medical professionals prefer the more precise term *opioid* for the substances that pharmacologically behave like *morphine,* the primary constituent of natural *opium*

Neuropathy: an abnormal and usually degenerative disorder of the nerves

Neutropenia: a blood disorder in which there is an abnormally low number of a particular type of white blood cell (a neutrophil), causing the affected person to be more prone to infection

Nosocomial infection: a hospital-acquired infection

NPO: a notation often made on a patient's chart meaning he is to receive "nothing by mouth;" he must avoid all food and beverage

Out-patient: one who receives treatment in a healthcare setting then goes elsewhere to recuperate

Palliative care: comfort care, care which aggressively relieves pain and other physical symptoms to give patients the highest quality of life possible at all stages of serious illness

Primary tumor: the original site of a person's cancer

Psychosis: a mental state characterized by a loss of contact with reality — the inability to tell what is real from what is imagined; persons may have hallucinations, delusions and personality changes; psychosis is a symptom of severe mental illness such as bipolar disorder, schizophrenia, and severe clinical depression

Radiation treatment: the use of high energy radiation to damage cancer cells and stop them from growing and dividing

Religion: a specific system of beliefs concerning the supernatural, sacred or divine, and the moral codes, practices, rituals, values and institutions associated with such beliefs

Schizophrenia: a chronic, severe and debilitating mental illness; a psychotic disorder; a life-long disease that cannot be cured, but may be controlled with proper treatment

Secondary tumor: a tumor that develops as a result of metastasis, spreading beyond the original, primary cancer

Spirituality: encompasses a person's sense of meaning and purpose in life, and can also include a relationship to a higher power or energy that gives life meaning

Suffering: the emotional dimension of extended discomfort and an indication that something is seriously wrong

Tumor: an abnormal overgrowth of cells, abnormal tissue swelling or a mass that may be either benign or malignant

Wonder: awe-inspiring, astounding, or marvelous

About the Authors

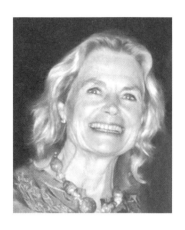

Geraldine Herbert

Geraldine Herbert, founder and director of The Creative Center: Arts in Healthcare, is a pioneer in the field of arts in healthcare. In 1994, she founded The Creative Center, a non-profit organization in New York, on the belief that people are more than their disease. Offering art and artmaking to children and adults with cancer and other chronic illnesses, Creative Center artists help alleviate anxiety, fear and boredom that are often part of the diagnosis and treatment process while helping them discover their own creative resources. *Art has a limitless capacity to energize our spirits.*

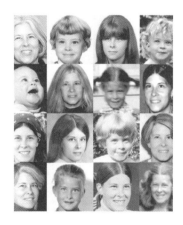

Jane Waggoner Deschner

In addition to creating and exhibiting her own artwork utilizing photography and the computer, she works as a consultant for arts in healthcare projects and programs; curator; teacher; organizer of large public art projects; and free-lancer in advertising, editing, writing, publishing and graphic design. She earned her Master of Fine Arts in Visual Art from Vermont College in February 2002. *It's a wonder to me that the arts are not a part of every human's day-to-day life experience — a photo or tune or poem can change the way we perceive and value even the most mundane details of our lives.*

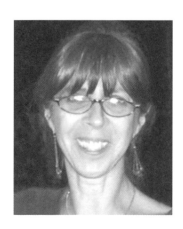

Robin Glazer

Robin Glazer is the art director of The Creative Center. A painter, printmaker and art educator, she is *dedicated to bringing art to people who might otherwise never experience the creative process.* A thirteen-year cancer survivor herself, Robin has helped develop numerous programs including a free-of-charge workshop program, a gallery and slide registry that features the artwork of artists living with illness, and the nationally acclaimed Creative Center Artist-In-Residence Program that is expanding to hospitals, hospices and healthcare facilities around the U.S.